Praise for Sharon's
SHADOW WORK

★★★★★

"I wish I knew how much magic I'd get after signing up. The decision alone caused a shift in perspective. I was so scared about the amount I'm spending on coaching with Sharon but it was unnecessary. I wish I had signed up sooner! If you feel the pull, then it means "Yes, go for it!" Trust that pull. Be prepared for the magic contained in working with Sharon. "Awakening" the knowing within and connecting to that inner higher self. There are inner shifts that cause ripple effects and long term results. – EDEN CARPEDIEM

★★★★★

"Sharon's coaching was life-changing, and critical to me feeling peaceful, powerful, and whole! Sharon's 1-1 NLP coaching, online courses, and meditations helped me amplify my true voice - the soft voice within. She helped me shed anxiety around self-worth, shift beliefs blocking me from financial abundance, and let go of fear about stepping into my power. I no longer feel alone, and I have given myself permission to receive all the abundance that is flowing toward me!" – CANDACE SUAVE

★★★★★

"Sharon not only helped me transform in such a short period of time but empowered me to be able to continue the work on my own. I live every day fearlessly and unapologetic. I make my own decisions and not from my own mind's chatter or from fear and conditioning but from my truest self." – EMANUELA ELIAS

★★★★★

"Working with Sharon pushed me to do, feel, and think about things in ways I never had before, which has literally changed my life. Sharon, you helped me change my outlook from timid to confident, fearful to empowered, dark thoughts into light-filled life. I am forever grateful to you. You have no idea the impact you had on me."
–LINDSAY LEE WILLIAMS

SHADOW WORK

GUIDEBOOK & JOURNAL

Copyright

For more information, email: sharon@sharonkirstin.com

ISBN: 978064583860290000

SHADOW WORK

GUIDEBOOK & JOURNAL

Rescue Your Inner Child From Trauma And
Transform Emotional Blockages Into
Manifestation Power

SHARON KIRSTIN

ALSO BY

SHARON KIRSTIN

THE ANSWERS WITHIN

Find Your Soul Purpose and
Ignite Your Hidden Superpowers

REVIEW & SHARE

Thank You For Being Here!

I really appreciate all of your feedback and
I love hearing what you have to say.

Would you please take two minutes now to **leave a helpful review on Amazon** and support others with their purchase decision?

Share a picture or video of the book on Instagram or TikTok and get **20% off any course**.

DM @sharon_kirstin or care@sharonkirstin.com with your video/photo link to receive your special discount.

Thanks so much!

Sharon Kirstin

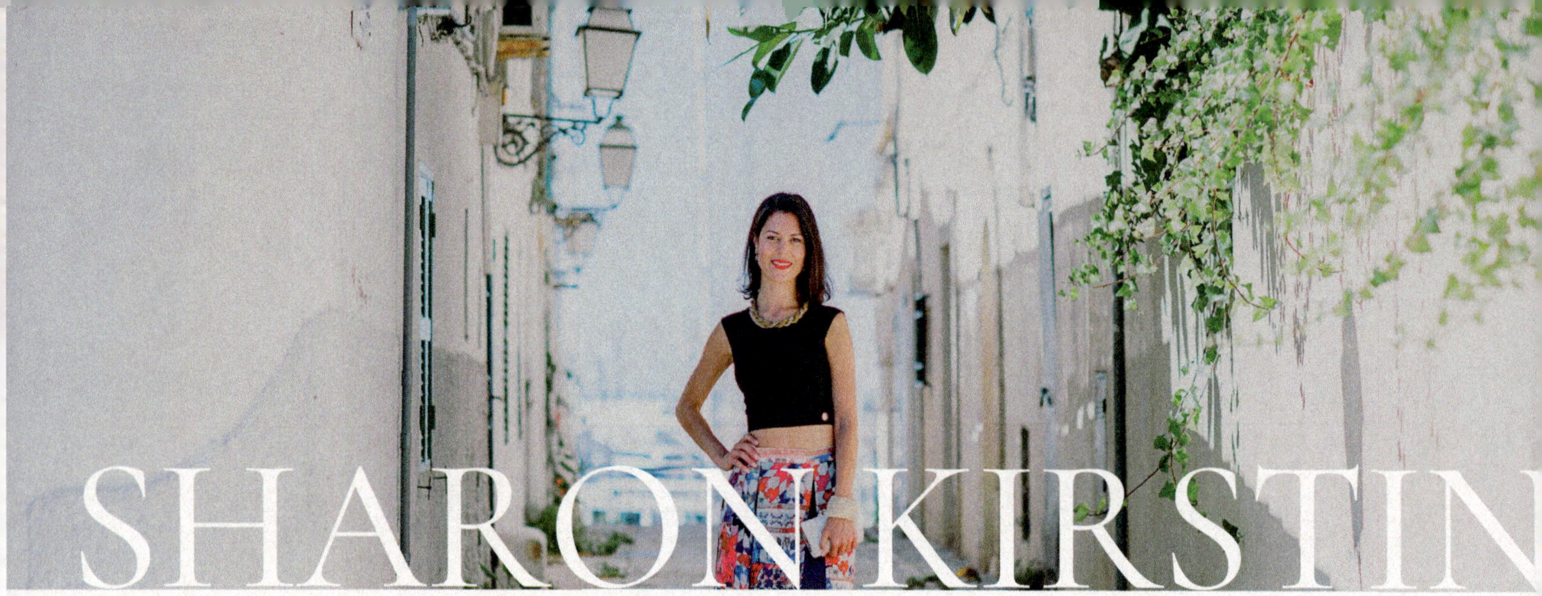

TRANSFORMATIONAL COACH

MINDSET | NLP | HYPNOSIS| SHADOW WORK

@SHARON_KIRSTIN
SHARONKIRSTIN.COM
@SHARON.KIRSTIN
SHARON KIRSTIN

Hi, I'm Sharon! As a Certified Master Coach and NLP Practitioner, I work with the unconscious mind – the Shadow Self – to help you heal your inner child and "reprogram" limiting beliefs and behaviors so that you can access all your inner resources to achieve your goals.

I'm a seeker of higher consciousness and obsessed with finding the fastest ways of unlocking our minds from limitations, control, and trauma so we can return to our God-given sovereignty. But I was a career junkie once! I helped build the most successful e-commerce company in Europe in a key role building and heading 4 departments.

Close to burnout and feeling a need to reconnect with my soul, I flew to the Indian Himalayas. In the mountains, I was touched by a transcending experience in meditation that led me onto a new path of helping others change their lives. I have been working with clients for over 12 years and keep expanding my knowledge...

Certifications:

German Diploma in Business
US Bachelor of Science in Business
Certified Master Business & Life Coach
Certified Master Angel Life Coach®
Quantum Healing Hypnosis Technique®
Beyond Quantum Healing®
Advanced ThetaHealing® Practitioner
Reiki Holy Fire 3® Level 2
Certified Sivananda Yoga Teacher
Emotional Freedom Technique Practitioner
Studies finishing in 2023: Clinical Hypnotherapy incl. Transpersonal Psychology

To Your Awakening

The journey to liberating our soul leads us to the dark side of our being and back. I honor you for being on this courageous path.

DEDICATION

CONTENTS

OUTLINE

CONTENTS

OUTLINE

What you CAN EXPECT

Shadow Work will guide you to shine a light onto inner aspects that are hiding in the shadows. You'll realize how these unconscious, hidden patterns have led you in your daily actions and choices without you realizing it. This awareness will create an opening, an opportunity, and a choice to change who you are at the core and reinvent yourself. Your whole world can change when you change your unconscious patterns, beliefs, and themes. It is deep work to excavate the parts of us we'd rather not face – they are hidden for a reason. Clearing the past will allow you to become truly present in your life without feeling held back due to the past or anxious about the future. This book can support you for many years and help you uncover the layers of your Shadow Self and return to the wholeness of Self.

Sharon Kirstin

Our demons will exert power over us from the safety of the shadows as long as we turn away and ignore them in fear.

The evolution of our consciousness guides us to face these shadows so we can 'enlighten' and transcend them.

When we heal these disowned parts we can reclaim oneness within ourselves and reinvent our world.

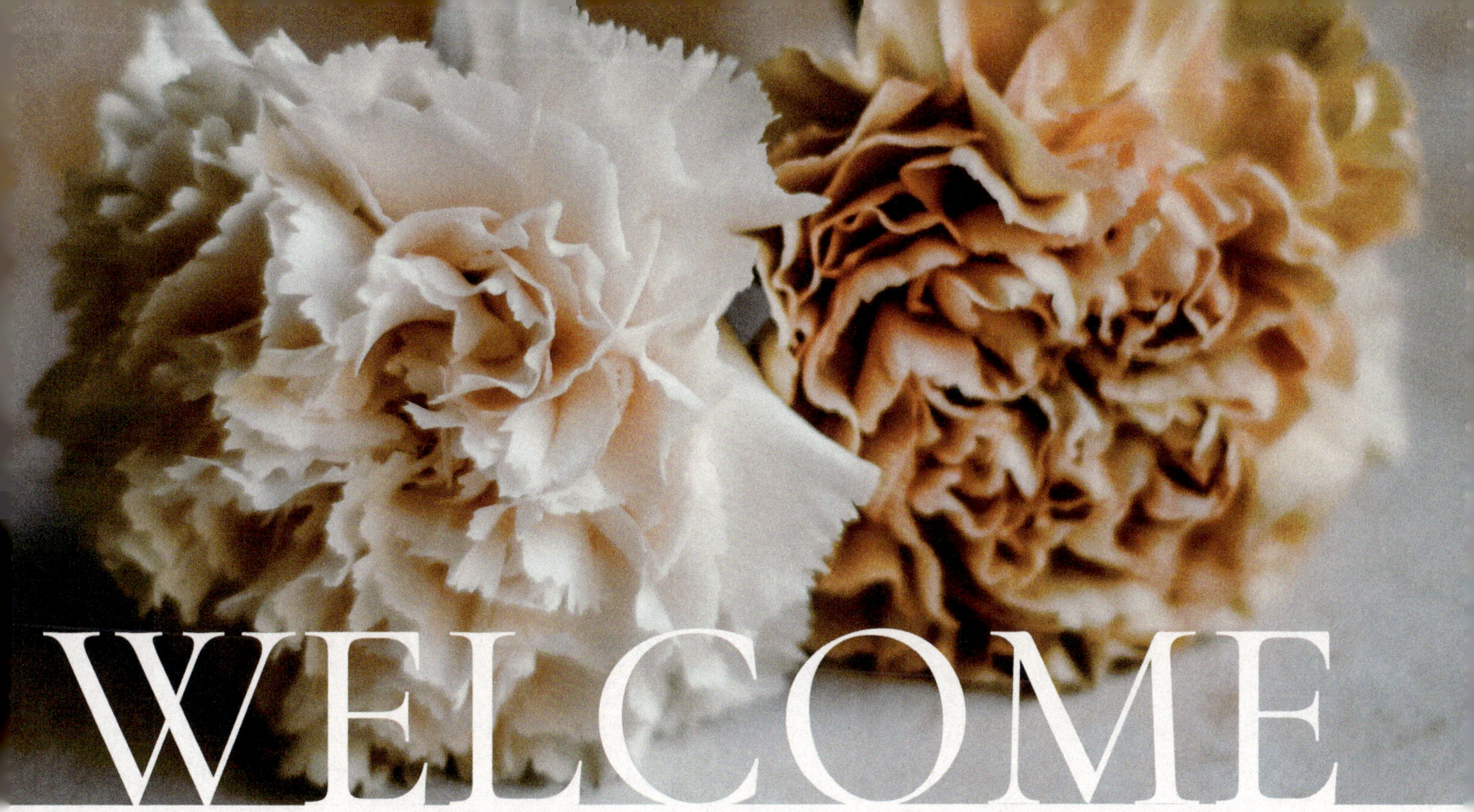

WELCOME

Shadow Work is a process of inner alchemy in which we bring unwanted parts to our conscious awareness for purification, healing, and integration so that we can find self-acceptance.

The paradoxical theory of change suggests that when people allow themselves to be fully and awarely in touch with who they currently are, change and growth then emerge as the inevitable and natural outcome of such contact and genuine self-knowledge. This is why we do Shadow Work. The word "shadow" can feel daunting, ominous, dark, and even evil. The popular "love and light" spirituality focuses only on positivity and "good vibes." Any negative emotions or experiences are disowned, gaslit, and pushed back into the subconscious. This has damaged the psyche and growth of many seekers because it further engrains the belief that we are not good enough and we need fixing. We miss a ripe opportunity for healing and growth. This becomes so toxic that we project our own demons onto others and can end up living in complete denial of our own shadows and their potential for our healing. The most important part of Shadow Work is that we own our "Shadow Self" without judgment. It's integral to hold our focus on empathy and understanding of our younger selves who had no choice but to live by these strategies to survive. Journaling, meditation, and contemplation of our own childhood conditioning, narratives, patterns, and cycles are powerful ways to break the old spells. Together, we will explore your shadow parts so you can return to your divine wholeness.

The Power of the Shadow

Our world is built on polarity. Shadow and light are two extremes of the same energy. When we do the work of bringing the shadow to light we increase our self-awareness. With it, we raise our consciousness and transcend the game of life.

In 2013 I worked in fashion e-commerce at one of the most successful tech startups in Berlin. I headed 4 departments that I had built from scratch.

On the surface, it looked like I had a corporate career so many strive for. While I enjoyed my job, I felt like something was missing in life.

I felt tortured by darkness within and it was hard for me to find joy in life. I felt like I was stuck in a black hole. Until a part of me urged me to reconnect with my soul - to connect with something "real" again.

Sitting in meditation in the Indian Himalayas I had a spiritual experience that changed me - I heard a voice say, "You created this life. You can recreate it." This moment forever shifted my perception of society, "their game", and the role I wanted to play in it.

I knew it was time to help others and contribute to a bigger awakening on the planet. But I kept running into my own insecurities, outdated behaviors, limiting beliefs, and coping strategies. I realized that starting a business is the best personal development program anyone can take.

I invested in coaches to help me get unstuck, aligned, and generate bigger profits. Unfortunately, none of them had the actual transformational tools to help me shift at a core level, feel different, take new action freely, and get new results.

I learned that most coaches can only share what worked for *them*. They had little skills and knowledge to understand the human psyche, trauma, motivation, and behavior. I also quickly realized the limitations of traditional therapy. Talking about the past without any resolution of surfacing emotions only pulled me into the past.

The surface-level advice from coaches and "talk sessions" with therapists didn't help me feel more empowered or free to pursue my goals. I still felt stuck. Maybe even more than before. I kept witnessing the same patterns and coping strategies play out and I started feeling fatigued by trying to "fix" myself.

It was a blessing in disguise because feeling stuck for so long made me deeply dedicated to finding answers. What I found is that if we want to create new results in life, if we want change, *we* need to change. We need to dive into the darkness of our being and heal the Shadow Self by bringing the pain from the past into our awareness. We can no longer turn a blind eye to childhood trauma, conditioning, and coping strategies because unless we face them, they will control us, and keep the results we desire at a distance.

I threw myself into learning about the human mind, our psyche, conditioning, trauma and so much more. After two business degrees from German and US American universities, I was a student again. I trained to be a master life and business coach, became a Neuro-linguistic programming practitioner, studied hypnotherapy, took energy healing courses, and so much more. By the time of writing this, I have spent over 10 years studying modalities and knowledge that can help you change your limiting beliefs and patterns quickly and gently so you can create the life that you deserve.

This is why you're holding this Shadow Work book in your hand. It is my contribution to your healing. It holds various concepts, insights, and prompts that are designed to help you dismantle your own demons within. In order for you to get unstuck and live your full potential self-acceptance is the key. Without it, you'll easily get misaligned and lured off-track by imposed desires from society that tell you what you "should" be, do, and have. It will be hard to know what is true for *you*.

Many of my clients can't even put into words what they look for when they sign up with me – they don't want to feel like "this" anymore. On the surface, they may want to leave corporate, start their own business, and find their purpose, but underneath it all, it's their soul calling them home. They may have had a spiritual awakening or a dark night of the soul.

A spiritual awakening is not a one-time event. We have many awakenings on our spiritual journey. Each one demands our courage and willingness to stare the truth straight in the eye, no matter how ugly, terrifying, or disturbing it is. This book has found you and you resonated with it. It is my deepest intention that the content and the journal prompts in this book will guide you to more wholeness and deeper self-love. Your soul guided you here for a reason.

xx Sharon Kirstin

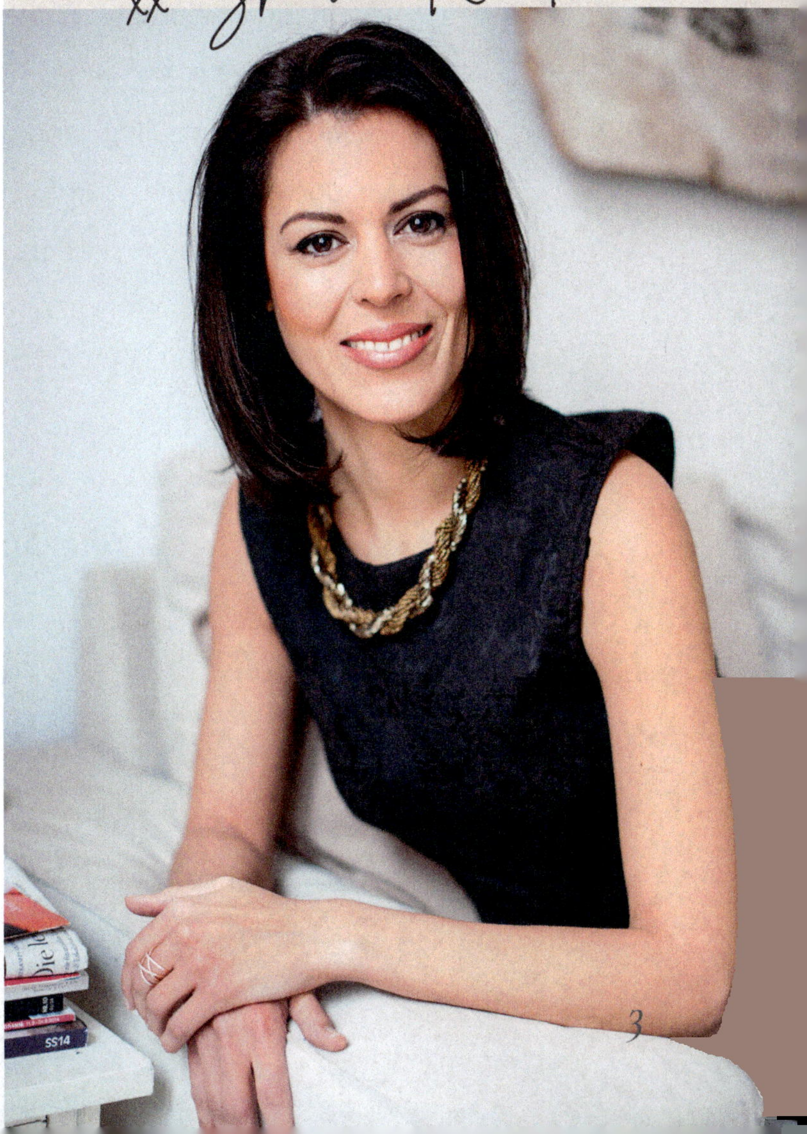

Your PROMISE

I promise myself that I will stay open to the process laid out in this book and will put my best efforts forward to bring awareness to my Shadow Self, how it has affected me, and how it still affects my life. I fully commit to my own progress, healing, and growth, even if it feels uncomfortable, painful, or tedious at times. I know I will be rewarded with gifts of healing, self-acceptance, and expanded consciousness.

Your Signature

01

WHAT IS SHADOW WORK?

01

A BRIEF HISTORY

Shadow Work Origins

The term "Shadow Work" was coined by Swiss psychiatrist and psychoanalyst Carl Gustav Jung in the 20th century. The central concept of Jungian psychology is individuation – the lifelong psychological process of differentiation of the Self out of the individual's conscious and unconscious elements.

According to Jung, a personality includes the persona, which is the personality that people show to the public, and the Shadow Self, which remains private or hidden.

The Shadow is an unconscious aspect of the personality that does not align with the ego ideal, leading the ego to resist and project the Shadow outward onto others. The Shadow forms out of our childhood attempts to adapt to cultural norms, expectations, and trauma. The Shadow becomes the Self's emotional blind spot. We can only see our Shadow as an external projection that shows up as the other – archetypes, metaphors, or personifications – within the collective unconscious.

This is why I mentioned before that the world around us will mirror our Shadow back to us until we become aware of it and do the healing work to "drop" it out of our field.

For Jung, it was the main task of human development to become aware of our true nature by realizing our conscious and unconscious parts.

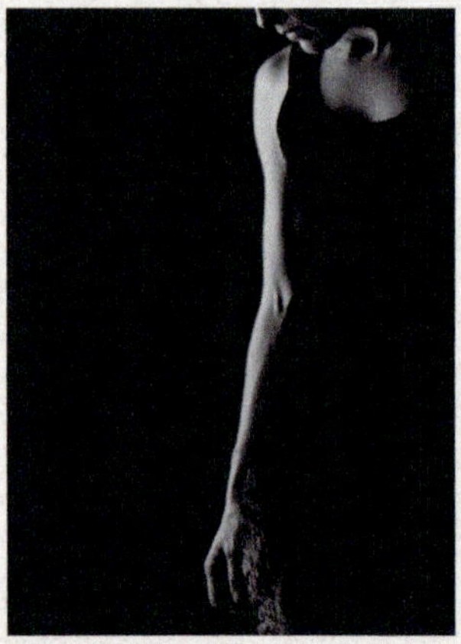

The Shadow Self is the collection of all parts of ourselves that we have deemed unworthy, wrong, and "less than". We have built a strong protection around these parts so much so that we can't perceive them in ourselves anymore. They need to be mirrored back to us by the collective.

Sharon

OVERVIEW

Jung's Model of the Psyche

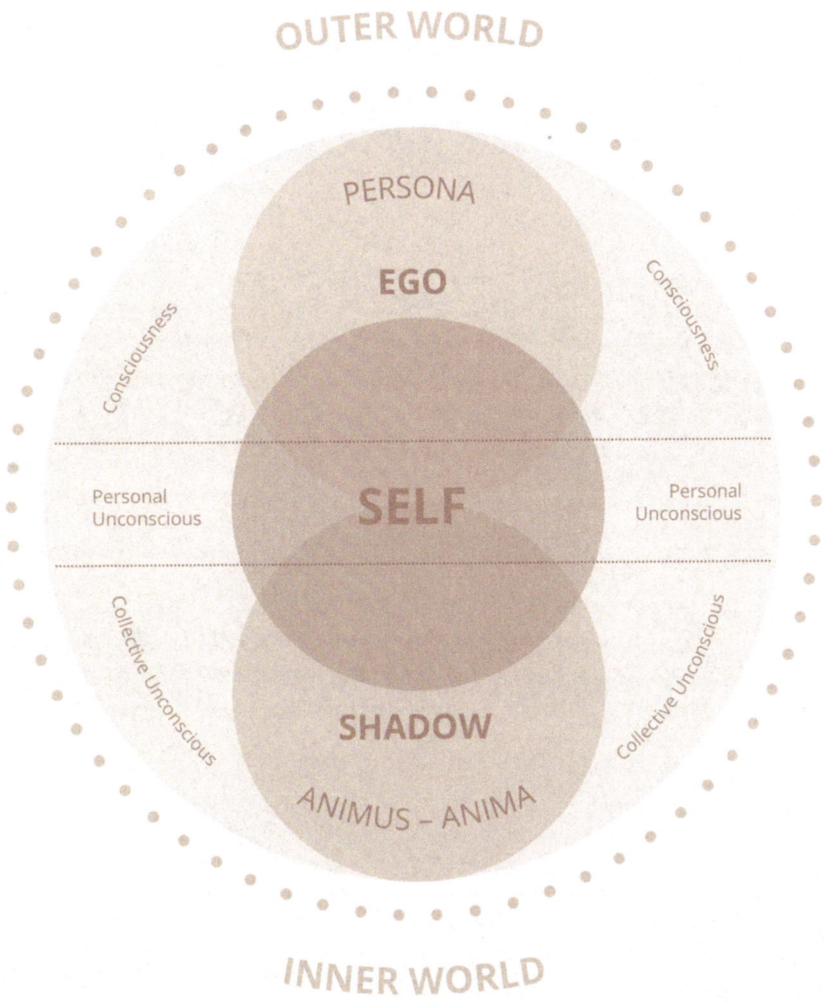

NOTES

THE PURPOSE

Shadow Work Benefits

01 *Higher Consciousness*

Self-development isn't about fixing what is "wrong" with us. It's about coming back to our divine wholeness. As we heal and embrace ourselves as who we are we expand our levels of compassion and oneness which elevates our consciousness.

02 *Increased Energy & Well-being*

Imagine carrying a backpack of heavy stones since childhood. Shadow Work helps us release this baggage and with it, gain new levels of energy and health. The body is a reflection of our inner self – the healing will be reflected in well-being.

03 *Improved Relationships*

The more we understand our triggers and the better we can communicate our needs the healthier our relationships become. Knowing ourselves deeply makes us emotionally available to see the other without our projections and accept them for who they are.

04 *Heightened Emotional Maturity*

Knowing ourselves, our triggers and needs will allow us to make new conscious choices about who we want to be. Not only will we be able to have less triggers but we'll have more compassion for other's needs and triggers as well.

05 *Expanded Intuition*

With so much heaviness gone and so much energy liberated, we become a vessel for inspiration and creativity. Our channels to a higher power get clarified and we can hear our inner guidance sounding through us. We are more connected.

Success Tips

01

TIP ONE

Compassion

Intent to hold yourself in loving compassion as you go through this Shadow Work process – no matter what you find or don't find. Shadow Work means working with the child parts of ourselves that we deemed unworthy and unlovable.

We are diving deep into the waters of our subconscious to dismantle patterns, themes, and beliefs that once served us but have outgrown their usefulness now that we are adults. Imagine yourself as your Child-Self as you go through this process. It is innocent and infinitely lovable. Treat your inner child with the love and care that you would any child.

Find a photo of yourself as a child and put it as your phone screensaver or on your mirror. This can help you remind yourself that you aren't working with an adult but with a hurting child that needed coping strategies to survive the pain it felt. Don't beat yourself up about repeating a pattern or "not getting it" sooner. You are here now and it couldn't have happened at any other time.

02

TIP TWO

Honesty

Practice radical honesty about your perceived shortcomings, failures, and those aspects of yourself you prefer no one to know about. Remember, we need to bring the hidden into the light of awareness in order to transform it and liberate you. It *will* get uncomfortable along the path. Hold yourself through these moments and intend for the projections to stop. Shadow Work is a brave act of radical honesty so that you can free yourself from the shackles of the past. Be willing to do whatever it takes.

03

TIP THREE

Curiosity

Be curious about why you do the things you do. Ask more and better questions about your motivations, needs, and results. Curiosity is an open, light-hearted energy that will serve you well to discover new aspects of yourself without judgment.

Success Tips

04

TIP FOUR

Non-Judgment

We're not going to play the "blame game." Passing blame onto others for who we are now means giving away our power and we lose our ability to transform and change. We are not what happened to us in the past, we are who we choose to be now. We are in charge of our lives. We can put in the work to reprogram our unconscious mind and bring healing to our shadow parts.

Generally, our caregivers had good intentions and did what they could with the internal and external resources they had available at the time. With time you will find that even if people mean well and they have our best interest at heart they may lack resources to implement this in a way that supports you. They are also only a product of their childhoods. We all have experienced a certain level of loss of Self in childhood to adapt. That's okay. You're doing the work now. If you have experienced trauma or abusive parents please get professional help. When we face buried pain there is always a chance of being retraumatized by memories. You deserve help.

05

TIP FIVE

Awareness

Awareness is the ultimate key to your growth through Shadow Work. Be mindful of the projections you place on others and the world as a whole. Be mindful of your words and the narratives you keep repeating. Be aware of what patterns keep manifesting in front of you. Bring awareness to your triggers and reactions. This is where you'll find the gold for transformation.

06

TIP SIX

Document

Stay grounded and observe your triggers and themes with curiosity. Detach and document what you find – this book is laid out as a journal by design. Just like a dream slips from memory quickly after waking similarly our disowned parts want to stay out of our conscious awareness. Writing down your discoveries helps you track and understand the bigger picture of your patterns.

07

TIP SEVEN

Regulate Your Nervous System

Our body keeps the score of every experience in our lives. The difficult experiences that made us disown certain parts of ourselves were especially painful and intense. Your Shadow Work will take you back to those intense emotions so that you can process them and invite a new perspective. It is important for us to feel it to heal it. Our nervous systems get stuck in trauma responses – fight, flight, freeze, fawn – which weakens our range of available responses. We automatically and repeatedly react in the same ways to the same stimulus. Our body is stuck in that moment in the past. In order to increase the range of emotions that we have access to it helps to move through our emotions intentionally and bring regulate our nervous system intentionally. Here are a few suggestions to train and regulate your nervous system:

01

Breathe

When you feel emotionally activated follow this breath pattern: 4 – 6 – 8 Put one hand on your heart and the other on the belly. Inhale for the count of 4, hold for the count of 6, exhale for the count of 8 through pursed lips. The longer exhale will help calm your nervous system by activating your vagus nerve, the pursed lips create pressure on your vagus nerve to relax it.

02

Shake

Help your body regulate itself moving through tough emotions by shaking your arms and hands while lightly jumping up and down. Accompany this with strong exhales to push and shake the emotional energy out of your body tissues.

03

Ground

Walk barefoot on grass or hug a tree. Science proves that grounding reduces inflammation in the body because it saturates it with negative ions, also called antioxidants. This restores equilibrium in your body.

04 *Sing or hum*

Singing and humming stimulate the vagus nerve at the back of your skull. The yogic Bee's Breath stimulates the vagus nerve through its vibrations. Inhale through the nose and allow a long exhale while humming gently.

05 *Senses check-in*

This is an especially useful exercise when you feel anxiety because it will help you return to the present moment. Focus on your 5 senses:

1. What are 5 things you can see right now?
2. What are 4 things you can hear right now?
3. What are 3 things you can feel right now?
4. What are 2 things you can smell right now?
5. What is 1 thing you can taste right now?

06 *Intimacy*

Acts of physical intimacy such as hugging, cuddling, and kissing are powerful ways to reset your nervous system. A level of safety with the other person is required for this exercise. The minimum time to reset is 5 minutes, an hour is even better.

07 *Exercise*

Physical exercise is a great help to reset your nervous system when you feel activated and to strengthen it overall. Vigorous exercise like HIIT training works just as much as gentle practices like Qi-Gong. Choose what works for you. The best exercise is the one you *actually* do!

02

PATTERNS & THEMES

02

Transcendence

"How do you find a lion that has swallowed you?" Carl Jung

What if all this time you thought you are "that" person but you are not? That "stuck", "self-doubting", "self-critical" or "depressed" person. What label do you give yourself, even if only in the privacy of your own mind? Think about it for a moment. What if this label isn't you and instead it's a symptom of the past?

Is it possible that you've been motivated and directed by an unknown force within? Unbeknownst to yourself? A hidden force that had you replay the past over and over with different people, in different situations, and different environments but still it is the same pattern? Many people notice that they date the same partner just in different bodies over and over.

Why would this happen? Why would we experience a similar kind of pain again and again?

The most beautiful perspective I can offer you to explain it is this: a universal force resides within you and all around you that is so infinitely loving that it wants you to heal. But it has only one way of communicating – reflection. One of the hermetic laws states "as within so without." This force uses this universal law to bring what is inside you in front of you so that you are able to observe it.

Everything in life is a reflection of yourself. And so this loving force externalizes your shadow, the hidden parts within, so that you can heal these parts of you. It allows you to become aware of the wound that created the pattern and find resolution in the now.

Conditioning

Imagine for a moment that we were computers. A computer needs an operating system on which "programs" run to execute certain tasks. We are born with an operating system, our consciousness, but no programs. As humans, we receive the bulk of our life programming before the age of 7. This is the time when our little brains operate in theta brainwave state. This is an open, hypnotic type of awareness. Since we have no ability to reject what comes into us we take it all in like a sponge with zero filters.

At age 7, the "critical factor" closes, the programming "drops" into our subconscious and we execute these programs without conscious awareness.
Much of what we believe about ourselves, the world, and our place in it, has its roots in this childhood conditioning.

Everyone carries a shadow, and the less it is embodied in the individual's conscious life, the blacker and denser it is. – C. Jung

Further conditioning takes place after that until we're adults but we move into a different brainwave state that does allow us to question and reject suggestions. But we live in a world of devices nowadays that are hypnotic and addictive by nature. Our inner sovereignty is constantly under attack with suggestions about looks, money, lifestyle, and more. But this is a topic for another time. For now, it's important to know that during our childhood, and especially in the first 7 years of our life, we receive the "programming" or conditioning that we use as adults.

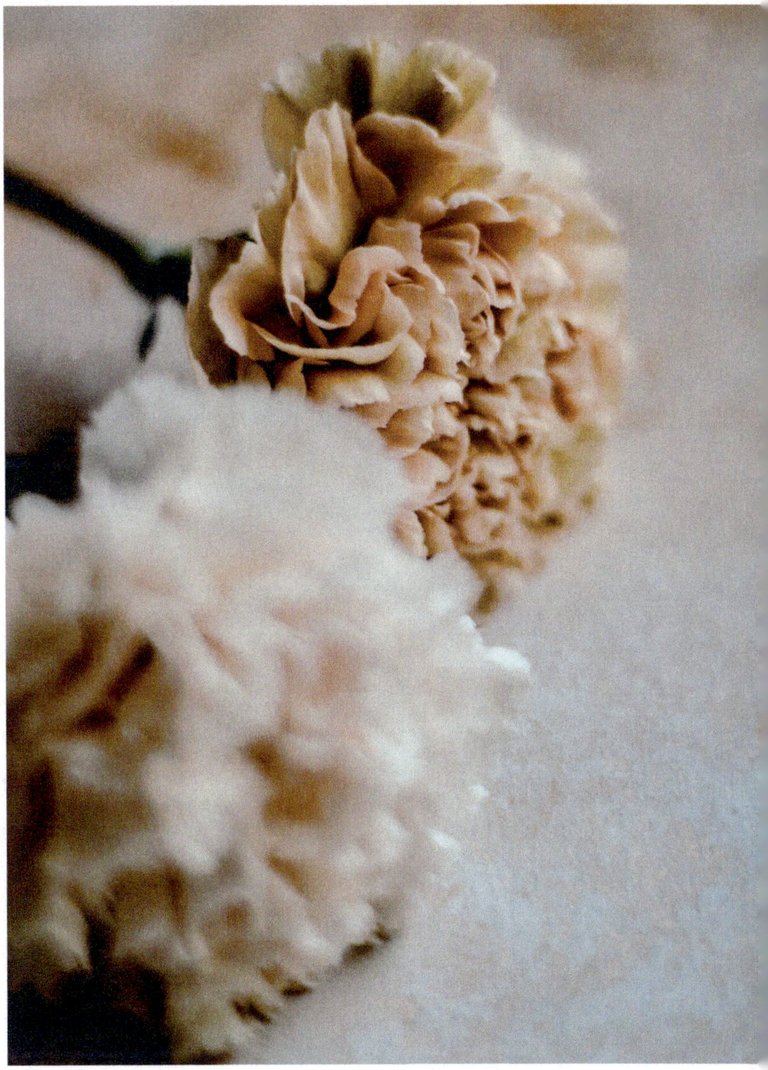

Survival

This childhood conditioning can be empowering or disempowering. Think of a program "The world is a safe place" versus "The world isn't safe." How different would these two people live, act and thus experience the world? Working with many clients over the last 10+ years I've seen two root causes for disempowering patterns (or shadows) that yearn for healing - trauma and self-abandonment. Undoubtedly these two can go together and often do, but not always.

As young children, we come up with strategies to survive by staying connected to and loved by our caregivers. Their love and care ensure our survival. So when we are in a situation where the loving connection with them is jeopardized we have two choices - either abandon the connection with them (and potentially die) or abandon the connection to ourselves (and survive). When parents create disconnection through criticism, neglect, absence, etc. our Child-Self didn't stop loving our parents. We stopped loving ourselves. Read that again. The unfortunate truth that I see time and again with my clients is that even loved and nurtured children can have this self-abandonment wound. Small incidents that seem like nothing to an adult can be a big moment for a child where they make a lifelong choice about their worthiness. If you are a parent, don't worry and please don't beat yourself up. You did the best you could with what you had available. And so did your parents and their parents. If we really want to let the past go and heal we need to become the gentle observer that holds no judgment.

> *Shadow work is about making our unconscious conscious so that we can liberate ourselves from old patterns through the power of awareness.*

By default, we have these unhealed parts of ourselves unchecked in our subconscious. That's why we have coping strategies like addictions that can be further detrimental to our mental and physical health.

Emergence

At the core of who you are, you are healed and whole. My perspective is that you're not broken, you don't need fixing and you don't need to push yourself to become anyone. You are whole and all we'll do is peel the layers that have distorted the truth of this wholeness. Freeing you from the influence of these past experiences that are still affecting your energy, behaviors, mindset, and actions. These shadow parts are wounded and hidden in the subconscious. Through the reflections from people and experiences, they are trying to show you that they are ready to be alchemized from pain into power so that you can embody a new way of being. And then the world can move from reflecting your suppressed pain to reflecting back to you this new self-acceptance and wholeness within you. You will manifest a completely different life.

This book is the door that, if you choose to open it, will lead you back to your wholeness that was lost as you learned to navigate this planet. But there is no transformation without awareness. We need to see it to change it. We need to feel it to heal it.

Often we are afraid of re-feeling the oceans of pain that once created our Shadow Self. We may have fail-safes in place to protect ourselves from seeing and feeling it. That's when we project onto others that they are the problem, the world isn't fair to us or we are the victim. It's *your* choice to take responsibility for your healing and positive change in your life. It's not your fault what has happened to you in the past but it is your responsibility what you do with it now. This book gives you the knowledge and self-inquiry tools to start reclaiming the innocence and power that was lost. You can take back charge of your life. It's a choice. Now is a chance to retell your story from a different perspective. You can change the meaning of everything in your life and regain your power.

Schemas & Early Strategies

Before we talk about what Shadow Work is and how we practice it, first, I need to tell you *why* it is such a powerful healing tool. You need to understand *how* and *why* you have become who you are now so that this awareness can give you a choice to continue or stop limiting patterns, beliefs, and behaviors. We'll need to dip our toes into aspects of Psychology and Neuro-Linguistic Programming for this.

Let me introduce you to something called, Schema Therapy (ST). It is an integrative approach that brings together elements from cognitive behavioral therapy, attachment theory, Gestalt therapy, and experiential therapies. It was introduced by Jeff Young in 1990. The most basic concept in Schema Therapy is an "Early Maladaptive Schema."

We can define schemas as: “broad, pervasive themes regarding oneself and one’s relationship with others, developed during childhood and elaborated throughout one’s lifetime, that are dysfunctional to a significant degree.”

That's a mouthful and basically means that "Early Maladaptive Schemas" began with something experienced in childhood, which felt damaging to us in some way. Subsequently, I will refer to these childhood "schemas" as "childhood conditioning", "strategies", or "programming".

We might have been abandoned, criticized, overprotected, emotionally or physically abused, excluded, or neglected. As a result, schemas (unconscious programs) developed that continue to *color* how we view ourselves, others, and the world. They still influence us.

A few examples of maladaptive schemas are:

CORE NEEDS

The child who didn't get its core needs met. Core emotional needs of every child include safety, predictability, praise, acceptance, nurturance, attunement, empathy, autonomy, validation of feelings and needs, fun, play.

TRAUMA

The child that was traumatized by a domineering, abusive, or highly critical caregiver.

CRITICAL VOICE

The child that has internalized the negative voice of a caregiver. This can happen by talking to the child in this way or the child observing a caregiver talk to themselves in this way.

OVER-DOING

The child that received too much of a good thing. It may have been overprotected, overindulged, or given excessive freedom without limits being set.

In order to survive and "deal with" stressful childhood experiences, that eventually create these schemas, we choose to adapt so we can feel *safe*. These adaptions become coping strategies that we unconsciously default to for the rest of our lives if we are exposed to a similar perceived loss of safety.

When a situation resembles our adopted schema or theme we no longer make a conscious choice about how we behave but we draw upon the strategies we've created in childhood that have successfully kept us safe. Common coping strategies are:

COPING STRATEGIES

- Aggression / Hostility
- Manipulation / Exploitation
- Dominance
- Overcompensation / Recognition-Seeking
- Stimulation-Seeking / Impulsivity
- Substance Abuse
- Compliance / Dependence
- Excessive Self-Reliance / Hyper-independence
- Compulsivity / Inhibition
- Psychological Withdrawal
- Social Isolation / Avoidance

If we lived through experiences that felt intense or like a threat to survival, we adopt even more powerful reactions. These are called *trauma responses* and there are four of them to choose from:

TRAUMA RESPONSES

FREEZE:
surrender and "play dead"

FIGHT:
overcompensate and attack

FLIGHT:
avoid the situation

FAWN:
appease the other to decharge the threat

These trauma responses manifest in everyday situations and look like triggers or reactions that are not proportional to the current situation. They are not proportional because they are a reflection of the past hurt, the initial wound. The pain is felt at the intensity of the initial childhood wound.

A shadow part within activates this trauma response to protect us from the same kind of pain we felt as children. Triggers are pure gold for our Shadow Work because they show us where we are still stuck in the past and see life through the filters and views of the past.

Neuro-linguistic Programming (NLP) will explain how this "coloring" or "filter" works in more detail in the upcoming pages.

Schemas are usually outside of our conscious awareness and live in our subconscious as part of our programming. We often only get information about such a schema, trauma, or program when we suddenly get triggered, react in extreme ways relative to the situation, and can't fully explain why we did.

These schemas or programs fight to stay alive. They distort our view of events in our lives in order to maintain the validity of their existence. They want to stay and so they hide in the shadows of our subconscious.

Are you starting to see why Shadow Work can be so powerful for changing the results we get in life? When we can become aware of our core programming and eliminate the distortions it creates in our lives, we regain choice.

In the following pages, you will find an overview of the 18 Schemas that psychologist Jeff Young has characterized. It is my hope that this overview will help you become more aware of what childhood program(s) you have adopted and how they are now playing out in your life.

We are only getting started so please bear with me as we lay the foundation for the deeper inner inquiry work that is to follow in later chapters.

NOTES

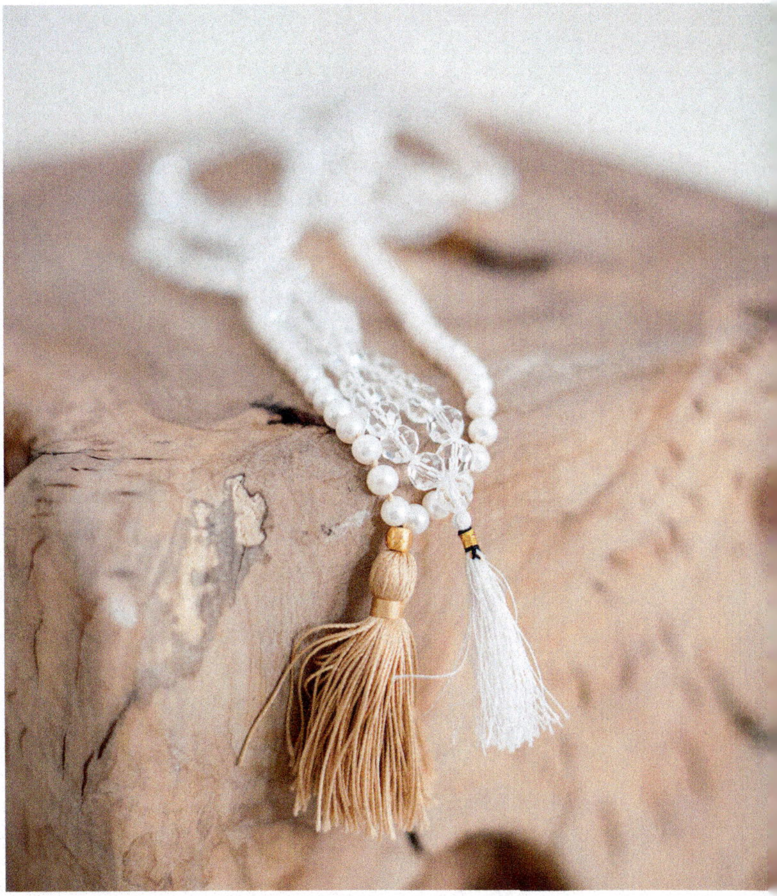

Disconnection & Rejection

by Jeff Young, Schema Therapy, 1990

01 *Abandonment & Instability*

The perceived instability or unreliability of those we rely on for support and connection. A sense that they will not be able to continue providing emotional support, connection, strength, or practical protection because they are emotionally unstable and unpredictable, unreliable, or erratically present. Fear of being abandoned for something better.

02 *Mistrust & Abuse*

The expectation that others will hurt, abuse, humiliate, cheat, lie, manipulate, or take advantage. A perception that the harm is intentional or the result of unjustified and extreme negligence. May include the sense that one always ends up being cheated relative to others or "getting the short end of the stick."

03 *Emotional Deprivation*

The expectation that one's desire for a normal degree of emotional support will not be adequately met by others. The 3 major forms are: 1) Deprivation of Nurturance: Absence of attention, affection, warmth, or companionship; 2) Deprivation of Empathy: Absence of understanding, listening, self-disclosure, or mutual sharing of feelings; 3) Deprivation of Protection: Absence of strength, direction, or guidance from others.

04 *Defectiveness & Shame*

The feeling that one is defective, bad, unwanted, inferior, or invalid in important respects; or that one would be unlovable to significant others if exposed. May involve hypersensitivity to criticism, rejection, and blame; self-consciousness, comparisons, and insecurity around others; or a sense of shame regarding one's perceived flaws. These flaws may be private (i.e selfishness, angry impulses, unacceptable sexual desires) or public (i.e. undesirable physical appearance, social awkwardness)

05 *Social Isolation & Alienation*

The feeling that one is isolated from the rest of the world, different from other people, and/or not part of any group or community.

Impaired Autonomy & Performance

06 Dependence & Incompetence

The belief that one is unable to handle one's everyday responsibilities in a competent manner, without considerable help from others (i.e. take care of oneself, solve daily problems, exercise good judgment, tackle new tasks, make good decisions). Often presents as helplessness.

07 Vulnerability to Harm or Illness

The exaggerated fear that imminent catastrophe will strike at any time and that one will be unable to prevent it. Fears focus on one or more of the following: 1) Medical Catastrophes: i.e. heart attacks, AIDS; 2) Emotional Catastrophes: i.e. going crazy; 3) External Catastrophes: i.e. elevators collapsing, victimized by criminals, airplane crashes.

08 Enmeshment & Undeveloped Self

An excessive emotional involvement and closeness with one or more significant others (often parents), at the expense of full individuation or normal social development. Often involves the belief that at least one of the enmeshed individuals cannot survive or be happy without the constant support of the other. May also include feelings of being smothered by, or fused with, others OR insufficient individual identity. Often experienced as a feeling of emptiness and floundering, having no direction, or in extreme cases questioning one's existence.

09 Failure

The belief that one has failed, will inevitably fail, or is fundamentally inadequate relative to one's peers, in areas of achievement (school, career, sports, etc.). Often involves beliefs that one is stupid, inept, untalented, ignorant, lower in status, less successful than others, etc.

Credit: Jeff Young, Schema Therapy, 1990

Impaired Limits

10

Entitlement & Grandiosity

The belief that one is superior to other people; entitled to special rights and privileges; or not bound by the rules of reciprocity that guide normal social interaction. Often involves insistence that one should be able to do or have whatever one wants, regardless of what is realistic, what others consider reasonable, or the cost to others; OR an exaggerated focus on superiority (i.e. being among the most successful, famous, wealthy) – in order to achieve power or control (not primarily for attention or approval). Sometimes includes excessive competitiveness toward, or domination of, others: asserting one's power, forcing one's point of view, or controlling the behavior of others in line with one's own desires – without empathy or concern for others' needs or feelings.

11

Insufficient Self-Control & Self-Discipline

Pervasive difficulty or refusal to exercise sufficient self-control and frustration tolerance to achieve one's personal goals, or to restrain the excessive expression of one's emotions and impulses. In its milder form, people present with an exaggerated emphasis on discomfort-avoidance: avoiding pain, conflict, confrontation, responsibility, or overexertion – at the expense of personal fulfillment, commitment, or integrity.

Credit: Jeff Young, Schema Therapy, 1990

Other-Directedness

12

Subjugation

An excessive surrendering of control to others because one feels coerced – usually to avoid anger, retaliation, or abandonment. The two major forms of subjugation are: 1) Subjugation of Needs: Suppression of one's preferences, decisions, and desires; 2) Subjugation of Emotions: Suppression of emotional expression, especially anger. Usually involves the perception that one's own desires, opinions, and feelings are not valid or important to others. Frequently presents as excessive compliance, combined with hypersensitivity to feeling trapped. Generally leads to a build-up of anger, manifested in maladaptive symptoms (i.e. passive-aggressive behavior, uncontrolled outbursts of temper, psychosomatic symptoms, withdrawal of affection, "acting out", substance abuse).

13

Self-Sacrifice

Excessive focus on voluntarily meeting the needs of others in daily situations, at the expense of one's own gratification. The most common reasons are: to prevent causing pain to others; to avoid guilt from feeling selfish; or to maintain the connection with others perceived as needy. Often results from an acute sensitivity to the pain of others. Sometimes leads to a sense that one's own needs are not being adequately met and to resentment of those who are taken care of. (Overlaps with concept of codependency.)

14

Approval- & Recognition Seeking

An excessive emphasis on gaining approval, recognition, or attention from other people, or fitting in, at the expense of developing a secure and true sense of self. One's sense of esteem is dependent primarily on the reactions of others rather than on one's own natural inclinations. Sometimes includes an overemphasis on status, appearance, social acceptance, money, or achievement – as means of gaining approval, admiration, or attention (not primarily for power or control). Frequently results in major life decisions that are inauthentic or unsatisfying; or in hypersensitivity to rejection.

Credit: Jeff Young, Schema Therapy, 1990

Over-Vigilance & Inhibition

15

Negativity & Pessimism

A pervasive, lifelong focus on the negative aspects of life (pain, death, loss, disappointment, conflict, guilt, resentment, unsolved problems, potential mistakes, betrayal, things that could go wrong, etc.) while minimizing or neglecting the positive/optimistic aspects. Usually includes an exaggerated expectation that things will eventually go seriously wrong, or that aspects of one's life that seem to be going well will ultimately fall apart. This is characterized by chronic worry, vigilance, complaining, or indecision. Usually involves an inordinate fear of making mistakes that might lead to personal disaster.

16

Emotional Inhibition

The excessive inhibition of spontaneous action, feeling, or communication – usually to avoid disapproval by others, feelings of shame, or losing control of one's impulses. The most common areas of inhibition involve 1) inhibition of anger & aggression; 2) inhibition of positive impulses (i.e. joy, affection, sexual excitement, play); 3) difficulty expressing vulnerability or communicating freely about one's feelings, needs, etc.; or 4) excessive emphasis on rationality while disregarding emotions.

17

Unrelenting Standards & Hyper-Criticalness

The underlying belief that one must strive to meet very high internalized standards of behavior and performance, usually to avoid criticism. Feelings of pressure or difficulty slowing down and hypercriticalness toward oneself and others. Must involve significant impairment in pleasure, relaxation, health, self-esteem, sense of accomplishment, or satisfying relationships. Unrelenting standards typically present as 1) perfectionism, inordinate attention to detail, or an underestimate of how good one's own performance is relative to the norm; 2) rigid rules and "shoulds" in many areas of life, incl. unrealistically high moral, ethical, cultural, or religious precepts; or 3) preoccupation with time & efficiency to be able to accomplish more.

18

Punitiveness

The belief that people should be harshly punished for making mistakes. Involves a tendency to be angry, intolerant, punitive, and impatient with people (including oneself) who do not meet one's expectations or standards. Difficulty forgiving mistakes in oneself or others, due to a reluctance to consider extenuating circumstances, allow for human imperfection, or empathize with feelings.

Credit: Jeff Young, Schema Therapy, 1990

Schema NOTES

Which schemas resonated with you? Write down the number and important notes.

Schema #

Schema #

Schema #

Schema #

Schema #

SUPPORT SHEET

The Feeling Wheel

As we move into self-inquiry through journaling, I want to share a resource with you that can help you pinpoint your emotions. The Feeling Wheel was designed by Gloria Willcox (1982) and is a great resource if you find it challenging to identify your emotions. I will often ask clients how something feels and they will use non-emotional words to describe a feeling, like "good" or "spacious." Often they have a "light-bulb" moment when they find the corresponding feeling. I hope this Feeling Wheel will be a useful resource on your Shadow Work journey.

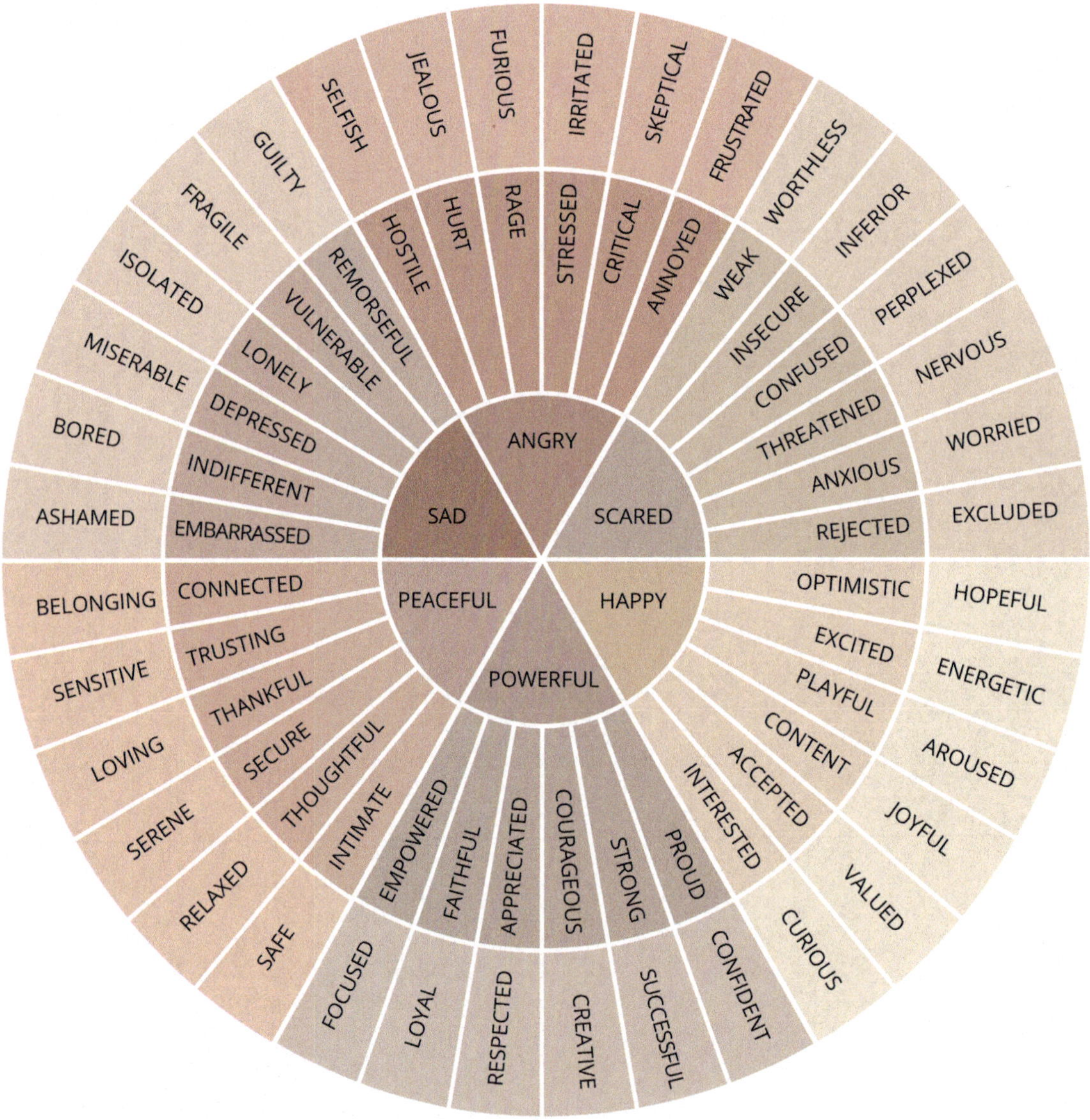

Journal PROMPTS

SCHEMA

1) Let's go deeper into each schema that resonated with you. How do I see this theme playing out in my life?

2) What memories do I have about this theme?

3) What bodily sensations, emotions or triggers do I have around this theme?

18 SCHEMAS

Journal PROMPTS

4) How does this theme negatively affect my relationships with others?

5) How does this theme negatively affect my relationships with myself?

6) What would my life look like without this theme? Who would I be? What kinds of relationships would I have?

18 SCHEMAS

Journal PROMPTS

7) How do I interpret situations in my life through the lens of this theme? Choose one or more significant situations and analyze how this theme may have played out.

8) Has this theme become a self-defeating life pattern for me? How so? Where can I see it?

9) How do I respond to situations that trigger this theme from childhood? What is my trauma response or coping strategy?

Journal PROMPTS

SCHEMA

1) If another schema resonated with you, let's journal about it here. How do I see this theme playing out in my life?

2) What memories do I have about this theme?

3) What bodily sensations, emotions or triggers do I have around this theme?

18 SCHEMAS

Journal PROMPTS

4) How does this theme negatively affect my relationships with others?

5) How does this theme negatively affect my relationships with myself?

6) What would my life look like without this theme? Who would I be? What kinds of relationships would I have?

18 SCHEMAS

Journal PROMPTS

7) How do I interpret situations in my life through the lens of this theme? Choose one or more significant situations and analyze how this theme may have played out.

8) Has this theme become a self-defeating life pattern for me? How so? Where can I see it?

9) How do I respond to situations that trigger this theme from childhood? What is my trauma response or coping strategy?

Journal PROMPTS

SCHEMA

1) If another schema resonated with you, let's journal about it here. How do I see this theme playing out in my life?

2) What memories do I have about this theme?

3) What bodily sensations, emotions or triggers do I have around this theme?

Journal PROMPTS

4) How does this theme negatively affect my relationships with others?

5) How does this theme negatively affect my relationships with myself?

6) What would my life look like without this theme? Who would I be? What kinds of relationships would I have?

18 SCHEMAS

Journal PROMPTS

7) How do I interpret situations in my life through the lens of this theme? Choose one or more significant situations and analyze how this theme may have played out.

8) Has this theme become a self-defeating life pattern for me? How so? Where can I see it?

9) How do I respond to situations that trigger this theme from childhood? What is my trauma response or coping strategy?

We constantly filter the world

At this point, you have an understanding of the kinds of themes we can adopt in childhood. You've also done self-awareness work to connect them to your own childhood, emotions, and patterns in daily life. You understand that we are little sponges until the age of 7 and it's likely we create maladaptive behaviors and themes during that time.

Before I introduce you to deeper Shadow Work and its alchemical power, I want to explain to you how our early childhood experiences can *color* and/or *filter* objective reality. What we perceive in our environment is never objective. It can never be.

Two people can observe the exact same situation but draw radically different conclusions from it. They paint their own subjective picture. How could this be? Shouldn't we all be able to observe a situation and agree about what happened and what it means?

You might have heard the story of the two brothers that grew up with a "no good" alcoholic father who ended up in jail. One brother grew up to be an alcoholic, kept getting in trouble with the law, and had many failed relationships. The other brother grew up to be a successful businessman with a beautiful family. As grown men each one of them was asked *why* they are the way they are. Both of them replied, "With this kind of a father, who else could I have become!" They lived through the same childhood but the meaning they gave those experiences and the conclusions they drew from them for their life were complete opposites.

Trauma isn't what happens to you, trauma is what happens inside of you as the result of the trauma.

What meaning did you give the experience? What did you make it mean about yourself, the world, and your place in it? Two people can live through the same trauma and it can affect them in completely different ways.

On the next page, I will show you the Neuro-Linguistic Programming (NLP) communication model. It explains how we interpret the world and how we process the constant and large amount of information that reaches our senses at every moment of the day.

It will help you understand why these themes (schemas) or conditioning we've discussed are important for us to become aware of. They are a big aspect of how we interpret the world and subsequently how we choose our behaviors. If we want to change our behavior this is an important aspect to understand.

Trauma isn't what happens to you, it's what happens inside of you as the result of the trauma.

OVERVIEW

NLP Information Model

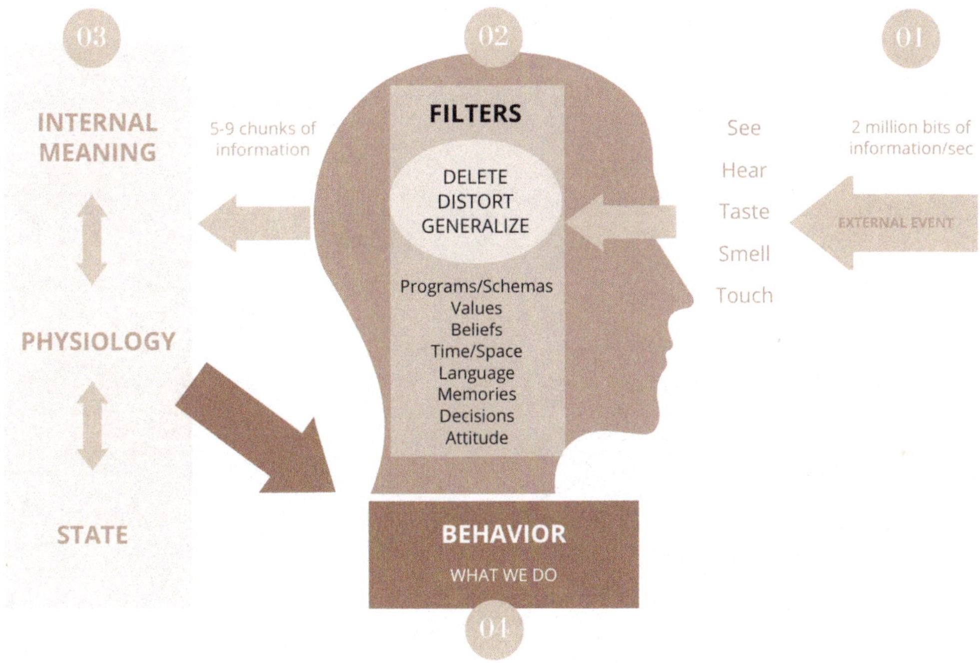

THE PROCESS

01 As we move through the world and have experiences, 2 million bits of information reach us per second. It's impossible to process all of it and so we...

02 ...filter the information based on our values, beliefs, programming, etc. When we filter we 1) delete 2) distort and/or 3) generalize the information we receive making it subjective versus objective reality.

03 At this step we have a few chunks of information left that get processed through our current emotional and physiological state, as well as our self-talk.

04 As a result we choose a behavior. Can you see how we can change our behavior if we change our filters – our programs, beliefs, etc – that filter and color our world in a certain perspective?

PATTERNS & THEMES

Journaling

REALIZATIONS

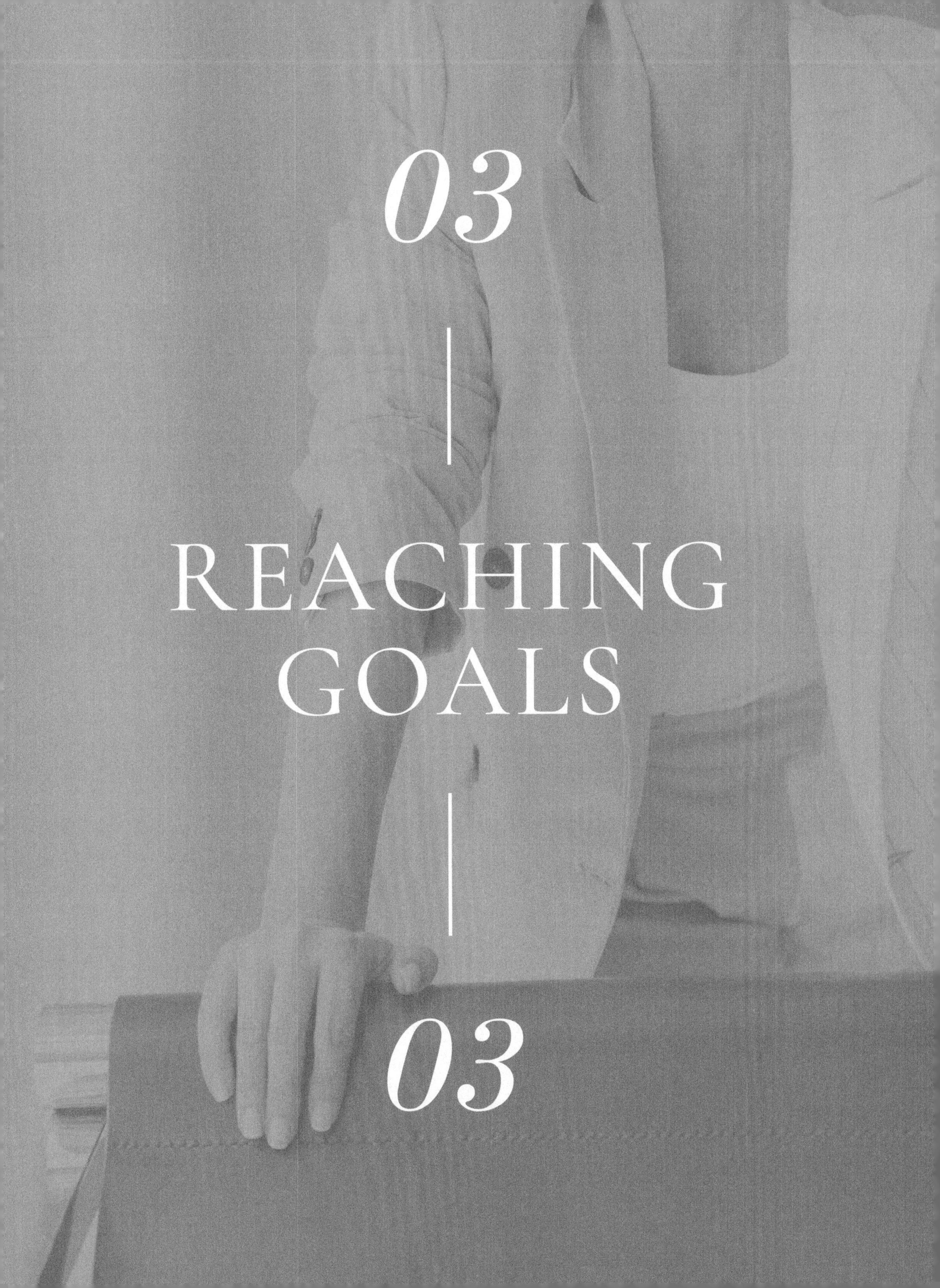

03

REACHING GOALS

03

Why goals alone don't work

As long as wounded parts of ourselves stay hidden in the shadows they have power over us. They are opposed to change because they don't feel safe with what is unknown. They drive us towards the safety of the known (no matter how destructive it is) and block us from changing in ways that feel like self-sabotage. It is a tight yet invisible grip.

Have you ever set a goal just to find yourself not following through in the moments when it counts? Think of the last goal you set. What happened in those decisive moments? When you ate that treat when you know you shouldn't? Stayed in bed instead of exercising? Went straight to sleep instead of meditating?

I like to explain to my clients that the conscious mind is the *Goal Setter* and our unconscious mind is the *Goal Getter*.

We usually know what we "should" do but we just don't do it. So why do we fail to reach our goals? Imagine having a bow and arrow. The Goal Setter would resemble aiming at the target, it is the vision. The Goal Getter is the correct arm and body posture to skillfully shoot the arrow so that it can reach the target. It is the execution, so to say. Unless both are aligned - your aim *and* posture - you won't be able to hit the target.

GOAL SETTER

With our conscious mind we choose a vision, a goal, that we want to reach.

GOAL GETTER

Our unconscious mind executes to manifest this goal. If the unconscious mind thinks it is not safe to take the relevant actions it will get in the way of achieving your goals.

THE SOLUTION

We need to bring the Goal Setter (conscious mind) and Goal Getter (unconscious mind) into harmony so that they work together. We do this through Shadow Work.

We need to bring the Goal Setter (visionary) and the Goal Getter (execution) into perfect synchronicity so that both are aligned with the same goal.

If not, we will have the Goal Getter (unconscious mind) living out misaligned patterns and behaviors that were learned in childhood. The coping mechanisms it learned in order to keep us safe so we can survive.

Instead of drawing upon our willpower and strength, in those moments the invisible grip can make us numb ourselves, run away, shut down, or put someone else's needs above our own.

In those moments it feels more comfortable to default to the known pattern instead of enduring the discomfort of new behavior. The good news is that with the right tools, we can bring healing to this wounded part so it will no longer sabotage us and get in the way. But first, we need to create awareness that offers us an important choice for change.

The opportunity in the Shadow Work we'll be doing is to bring resolution to these parts of ourselves that are stuck in the past, afraid to move forward.

We can help ourselves become whole again. We can give ourselves access to a bigger range of emotional recourses. We can calm our nervous system. We can access a greater capacity for taking risks.

And all this leads to being able to follow through on our goals from a place of clarity, self-love, resourcefulness, and strength.

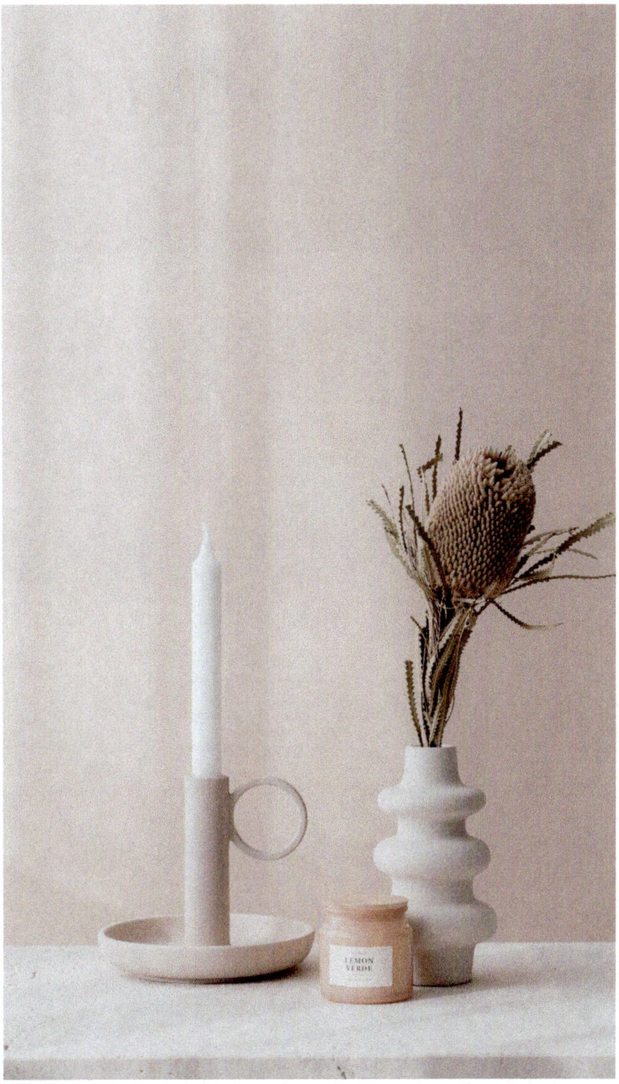

NOTES

Smart GOALS

S
Make it specific

What is your specific goal? Think numbers and dates, who, where, when, why and what.

M
Make it measurable

How will you measure the success of your goal? Your goals should include a quantity of 'how much' or 'how many'.

A
Make it attainable

What steps are you going to take? If you don't have time, supplies, or the right location, make adjustments to your methods and goals.

R
Make it relevant

What makes this goal worth working for? Make sure you know your why.

T
Make it timely

When is the deadline? Deadlines can motivate your efforts and prioritize the task above other distractions.

WORKSHEET

Goal Setter vs. Goal Getter

Use this worksheet to identify what gets in the way of progress. Use the top boxes to set your goal and identify your action steps. This is your Goal Setter, conscious mind. Use the bottom boxes to identify what gets in the way of your follow-through. This will give you clarity about what strategies and needs your Goal Getter, unconscious mind, has instead.

WHAT IS YOUR GOAL?

DEADLINE:

3 ACTION STEPS

01

02

03

WHAT GETS IN THE WAY?

CORE NEED MET:

LIMITING BELIEFS

01

02

03

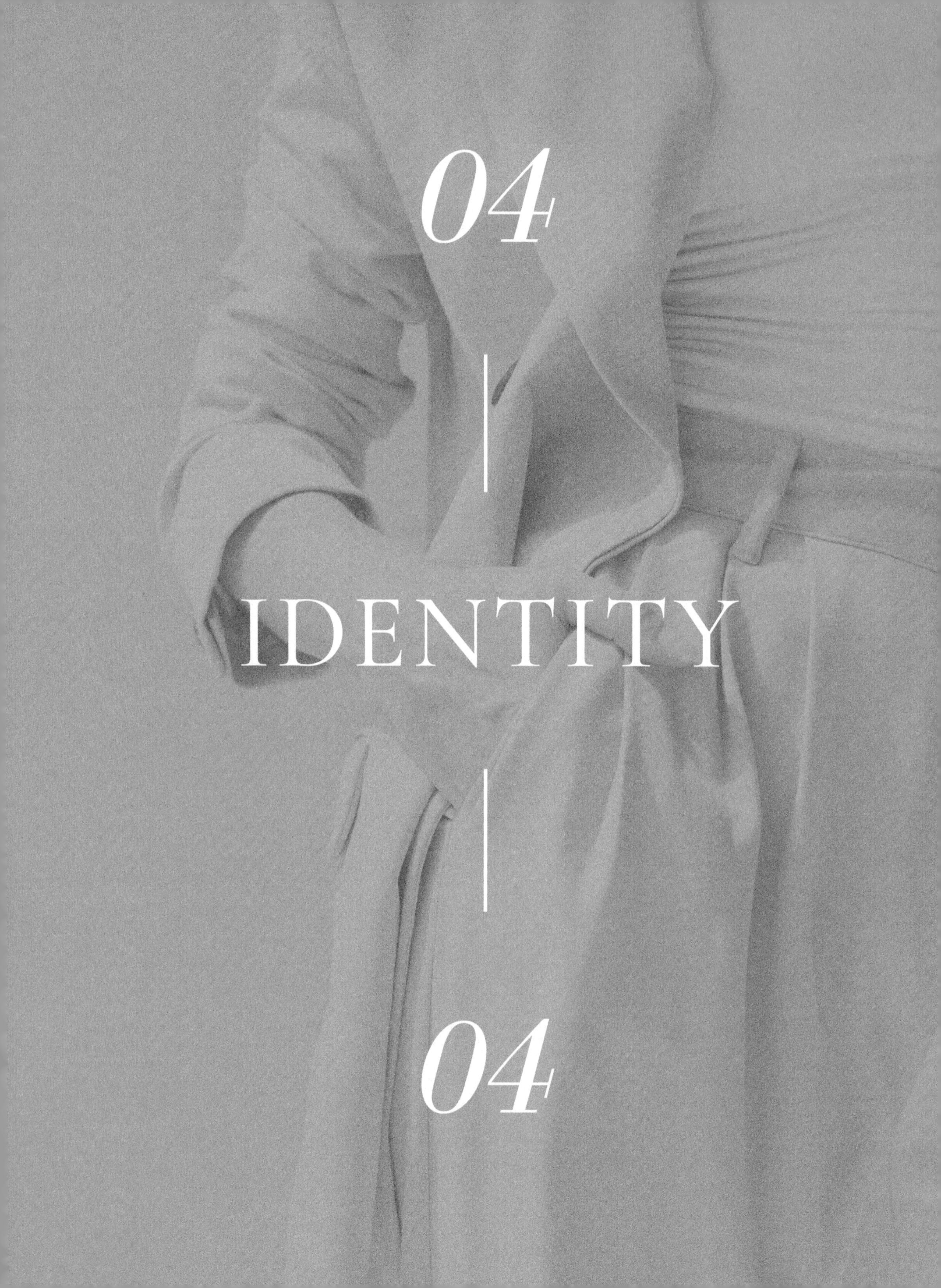

04

IDENTITY

04

CHAPTER 04
IDENTITY WORK

By now, it's probably dawning on you – our identity is mainly made up of our childhood *conditioning*. The experiences we've lived through and the meanings we've given these events in regard to ourselves and the world around us *still* has an effect on us. As you now know there are conscious and unconscious parts of our psyche. Our childhood conditioning is still the operating system that most of our decisions are based on. Our impulsive reactions and even our dreams and yearnings come from this unconscious part of our psyche. We like to imagine that we play a conscious part in our daily life but if we haven't questioned why we do things a certain way yet, we are still mainly operating as a product of our childhood conditioning.

I've explained this in Chapter 1, but I want to mention it again – until 7 years old, we are sponges. We are unable to reject what we see, feel, and are being told. We are being programmed by our surroundings into an identity that we will later accept as "who we are." We function much like little computers that once we're programmed to do a certain task we go on autopilot when we execute. Just think back to the first time you drove a car or

WORKSHEET

Hierarchy of Learning

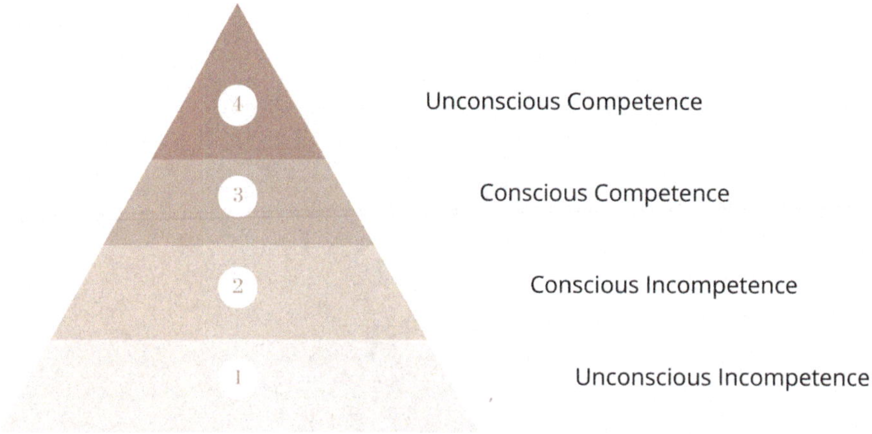

1

Unconscious Incompetence

This is the initial stage where we are unaware that we don't know. We may even deny the usefulness of a new skill. We must recognize our own incompetence, and the value of the new skill, before moving on to the next stage. How much time we spend in this stage depends on the intensity of pain we feel.

2

Conscious Incompetence

At this stage, we recognize our deficit and become willing to change. We want to learn because we see value in the new skill to overcome our deficit. Making mistakes is part of the learning process at this stage.

3

Conscious Competence

We understand or know how to do something but there is heavy conscious involvement in executing the new skill. Using the skill or knowledge requires concentration, and if it is broken, we lapse into incompetence.

4

Unconscious Competence

We've had so much practice with a skill that it has become "second nature" or "automatic". We can perform it easily. As a result, the skill can be performed while executing another task. We may be able to teach it to others.

did anything for the first time that you do daily now. At first, you had to consciously think of every single step. But when you get into a car now you do everything unconsciously. You don't consciously think about all the tasks that need to happen simultaneously. It has become "second nature" and you're on autopilot.

There are three main ways in which we get programmed:

1. Repetition
2. Emotional intensity (good or bad)
3. Theta Brainwaves

And once we are programmed we behave, think, and act on autopilot without our conscious involvement. I've added the "Hierarchy of Learning" scale for you because it shows you how to get the most out of your Shadow Work over time. But more importantly, it highlights an important fact: We are unconsciously competent at being who we are now. We've experienced all three kinds of programming to create our identity, especially in childhood. While we were in theta brainwave state we had emotionally intense experiences that often repeated themselves in various scenarios. And on top of this, we can't even remember it.

In childhood, the main messages we receive are about who we *should* be in order to fit into our parents' lives and society overall. Many of us weren't encouraged to live our truth but to behave in a way that doesn't disturb adults. During this innocent time, we're learning who we should be and are starting to lose the sacred connection to our inner Self.

NOTES

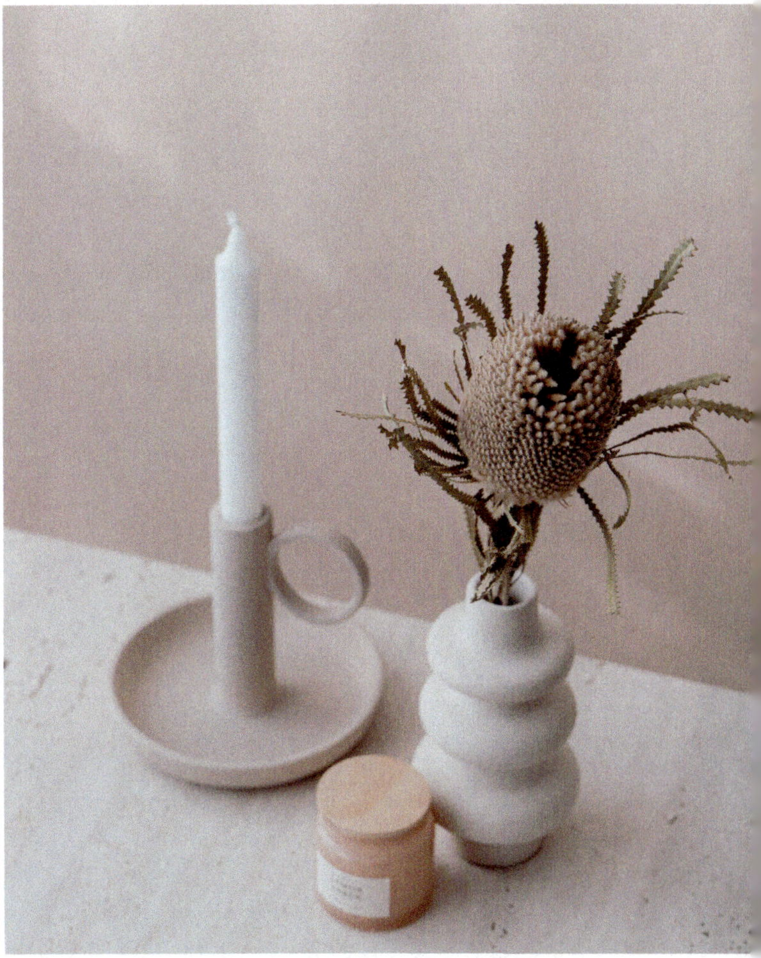

Journal PROMPTS

01 *Write down the repeated suggestions you have received as a child. What did your parents tell you to be? Common ones are, "Kids are seen, not heard." "You're not allowed to talk when adults speak."*

02 *Let's go further. Who did your parents tell you to be? Did you have to be quiet, clean, or helpful? What are some expectations your caregivers had of you?*

OVERVIEW

Identity Layers

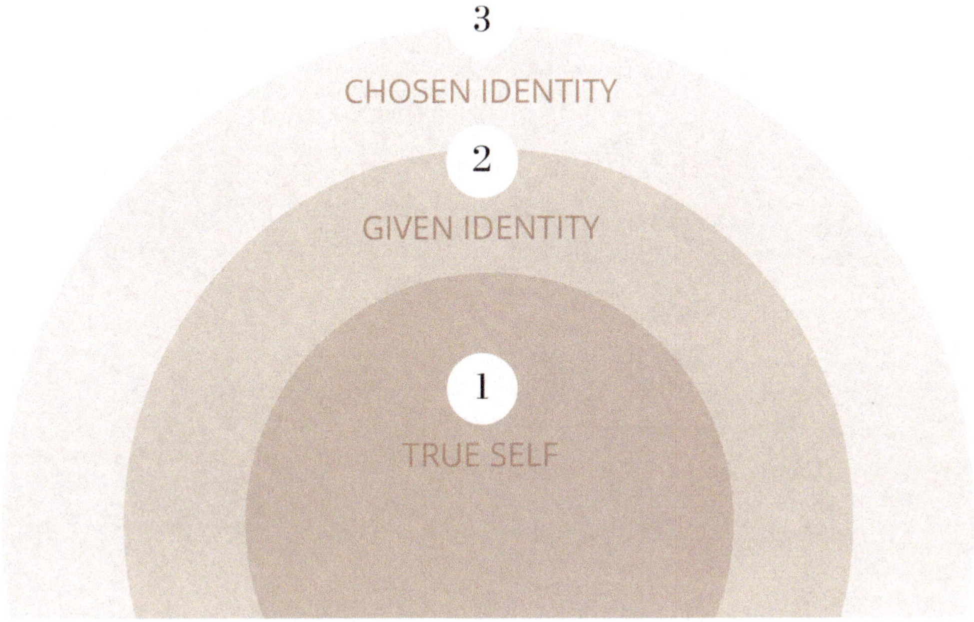

01
CORE

True Self

Our God-Given Identity with your talents, traits and characteristics that make us unique. At our core we are effortlessly connected to the infinite intelligence of the universe. We hear our intuition loud and clear and know what is right for us.

02
LAYER

Given Identity

In this layer we receive the conditioning in childhood about what are un/wanted behaviors from us, societal imprints, media, ethnicity/race, culture, location and opportunities but also traumatic experiences.

03
LAYER

Chosen Identity

This is where we move into shaping who we are through interests, things that we dedicate our time, attention and focus to. Basically, consciously learned behaviors through repetition and choice.

Influences on Identity

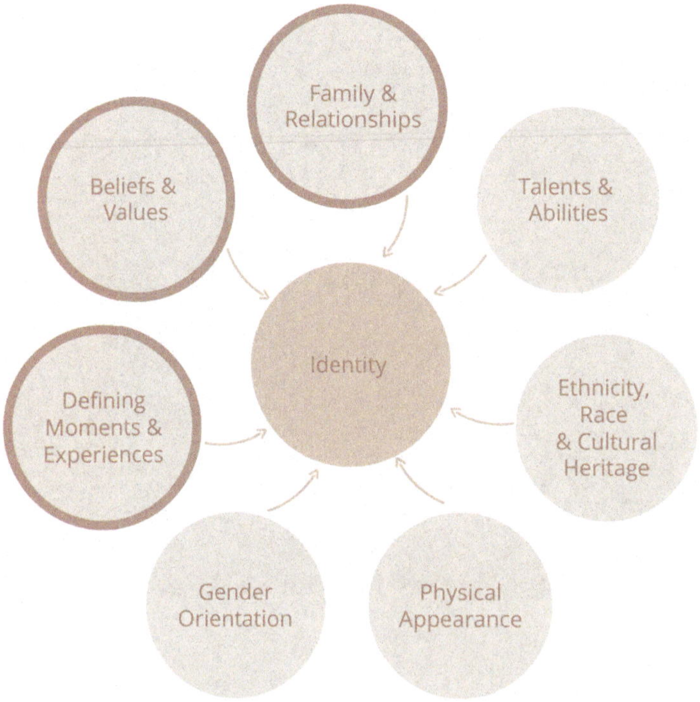

The Top Influences

The three main identity influences that we will look at through our Shadow Work are:

1. Beliefs & Values
2. Defining Moments & Experiences
3. Family & Relationships

Of course, all influences are entangled. We can't separate one influence from another because they all shape what we believe about ourselves and the world. For instance, our family has a huge impact on our beliefs and values. Just like our physical appearance or talents strongly influence what we believe about ourselves. Our main Shadow Work goal is to uncover the hidden beliefs and experiences that have left a lasting imprint that is *no longer serving us now that we're adults.*

Once we find the root cause of a belief – no matter whether its root lies in family conditioning, a traumatic experience, or our cultural imprinting – we can make empowering changes that lead us to better results in life.

Journal PROMPTS

01 *Describe who you are. Imagine yourself describing a new friend, but that new friend is you. What would you say about who you are? Think of character traits, behaviors, interests, routines, values, occupation, family and all the other influences from the page before.*

Journal PROMPTS

02 *Describe who you are within. Describe the aspects of you that no one ever gets to see. Think of emotions, hopes, fears, worries, insecurities, etc.*

03 *Describe who you are in public. How do you present yourself to the world? Describe the aspects that you show to others. How would they describe you?*

Journal PROMPTS

04 *List at least 5 aspects of you that you do not show others. What do you notice about them – is there an overarching "theme"? Something you don't want others to see and know?*

05 *Are there aspects of you that you try to "cover up" or hide from others? List each one and explain why you hide it. What do you notice, is there a "theme"?*

WORKSHEET

Expressing Your Identities

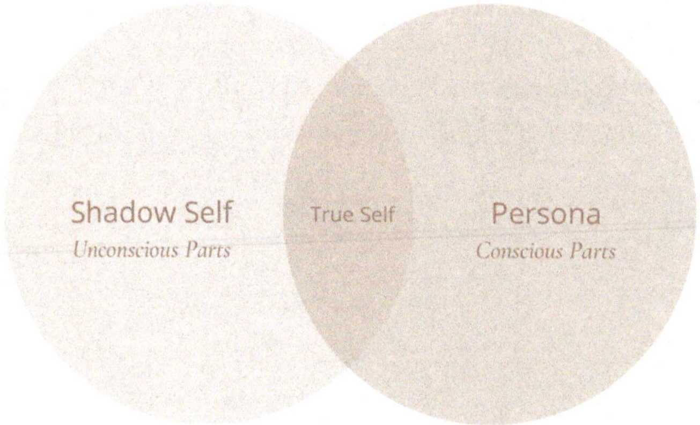

01

"Shadow Self" Identity

Describe this version of you:

02

"Persona" Identity

Describe this version of you:

03 *True Self*

How do these two versions of you differ – your Shadow Self and public Persona? Contemplate when you show which identity and why. When do you cover up your true self?

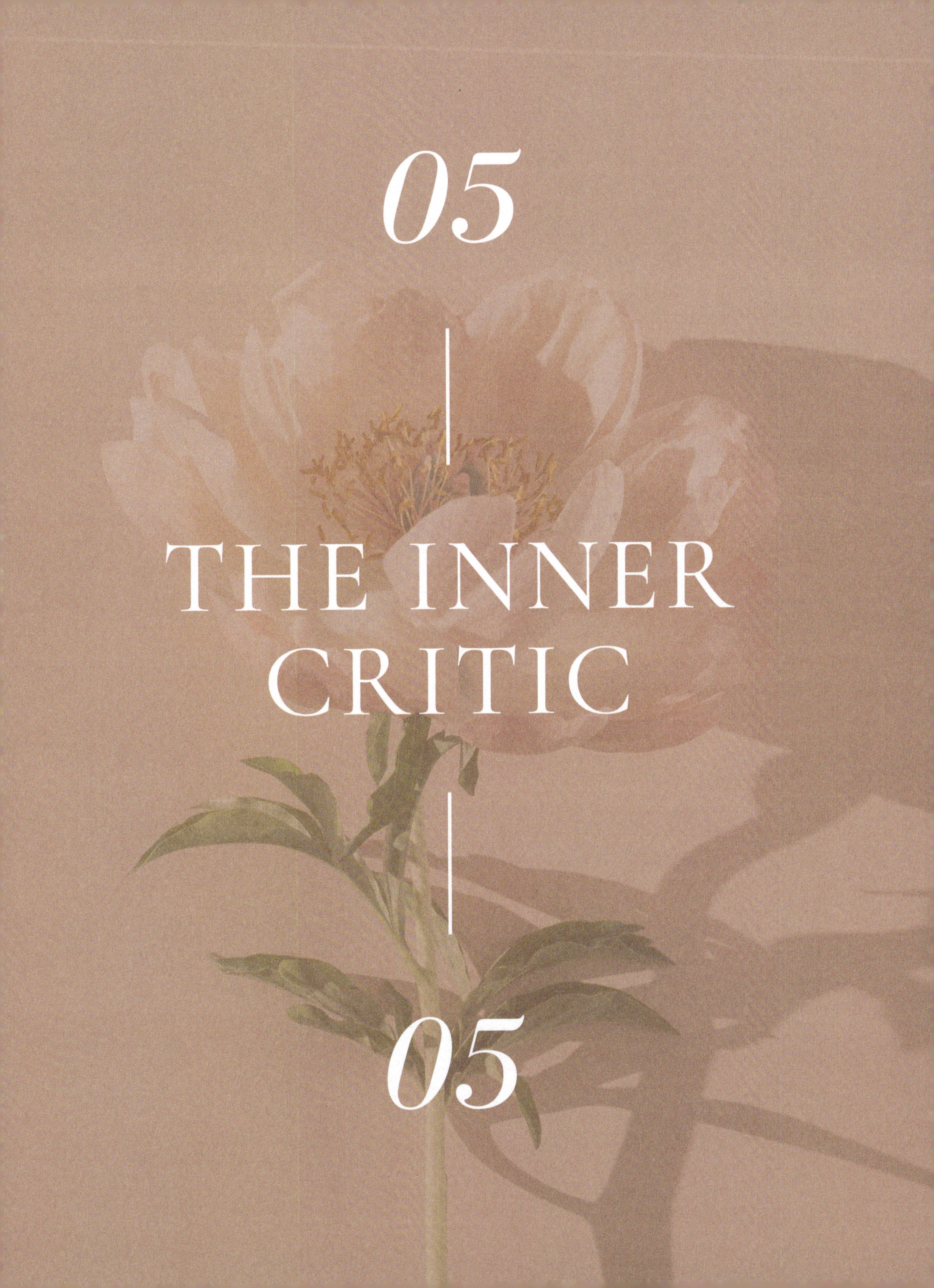

05

THE INNER CRITIC

05

chapter five

WHEN INNER DIALOGUE HURTS

Know that voice inside your head that says nasty things to and about you? It can make you afraid or put you down. It likes to second-guess your choices and relentlessly goes over what you did earlier to point out what you should've done differently. It's that nasty inner critic that tortures you from within your own mind.

The inner critic is a voice that we have adopted at some point in childhood. It usually belongs to a caregiver that either spoke to us in this way or we witnessed them talking to themselves or others in this way. The good news is – it's not ours so we can change it!

Let's shine the light of awareness on it in this chapter. And remember, trust the first answer you receive intuitively. The first answer comes from your unconscious mind, the second one is the edited version by the conscious mind. We want to make the unconscious conscious, so always trust the first answer, idea, or thought you receive.

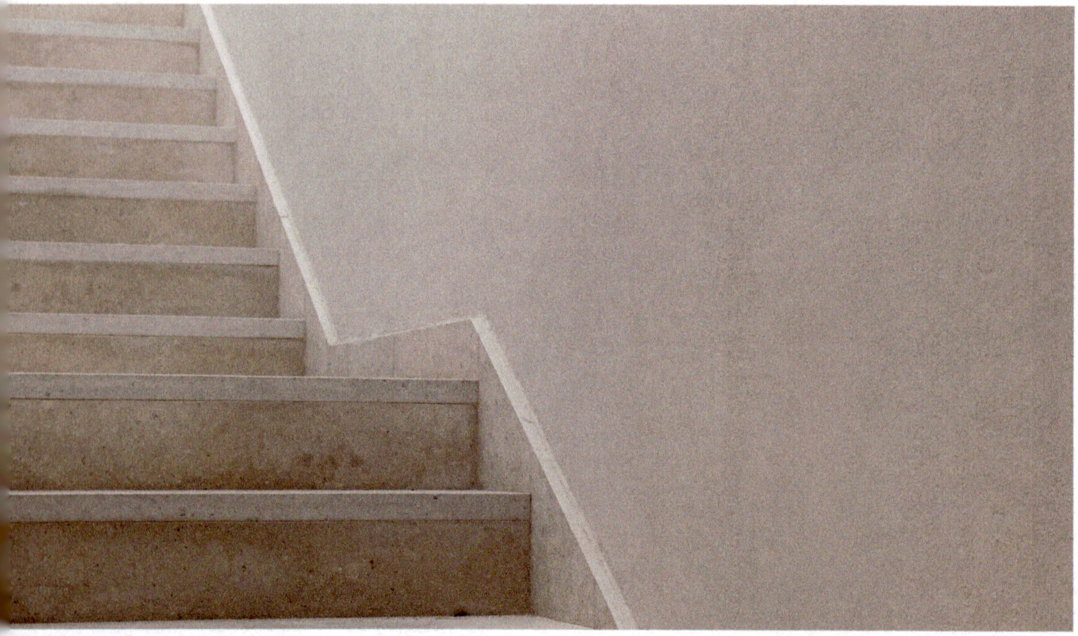

WORKSHEET

Identify Your Inner Critic

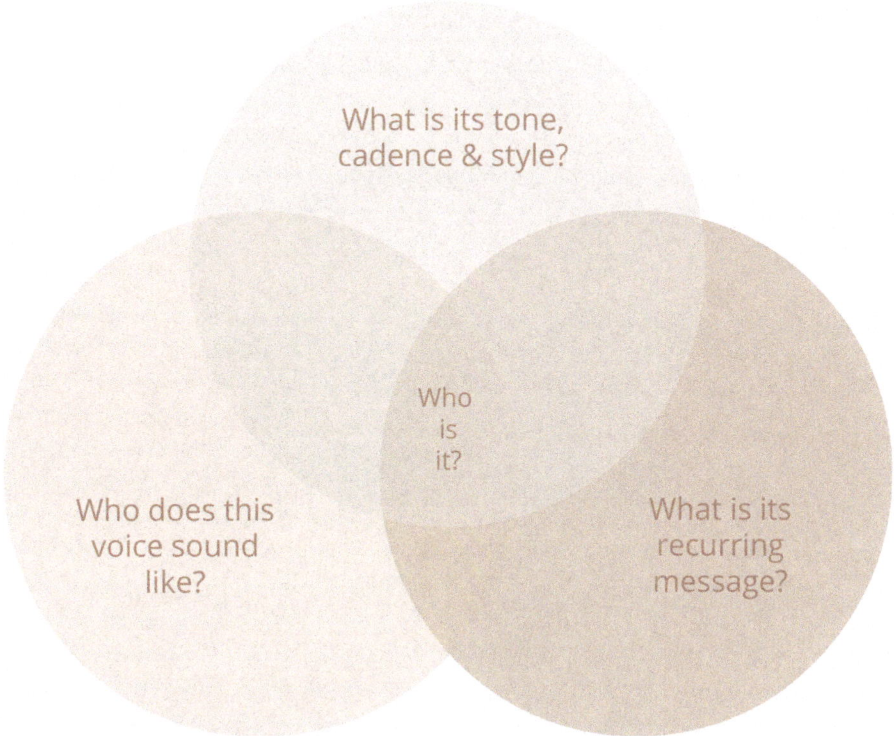

Our Inner Critic is often times the voice of one of our caregivers when we were a child. Unfortunately, criticism is internalized when we are young. When kids hear repeatedly what they are doing is wrong, they don't hear *what* they are *doing* is wrong. They hear, "I *am* wrong." Let's identify what caregiver's voice you have internalized. The tricky part is that over time the Inner Critic seems to sound like our own inner voice. But when we are vigilant and aware, we can find out who is really still criticizing us and change our inner narrative.

JOURNAL

Journal PROMPTS

01 *Think of a time when you made a mistake, what did your Inner Critic say to you? A helpful way to bring up relevant experiences is to let our unconscious mind present them to us. Read the question again and close your eyes, take a deep breath – what is the first incident that comes to mind?*

02 *And from a different angle – think of a time when your Inner Critic was very vocal and loud, what did it say?*

INNER CRITIC

Journal PROMPTS

03 *Think of a time when you felt insecure, what did it say?*

04 *Think of a time when you felt hopeless, what did it say then?*

05 *Think of a time when you worried, what did it make you afraid of?*

06 *Think of a time when you felt "found out about," what did it say?*

Journal PROMPTS

07 *What are the times your Inner Critic is the loudest? List 3 different kinds of situations.*

08 *Close your eyes, take a deep breath, and let your unconscious mind show you a memory of a time when your Inner Critic was very loud. What was happening and what did it say?*

09 *Now, read through your answers. Does your Inner Critic sound like someone you know? If you knew who your Inner Critic was, it would be...*

EXERCISE

Cartoon Character

For this exercise, we need two things: 1) a cartoon figure that you find so silly that you could never take what they say seriously, like the Roadrunner or Tweety, for instance. And 2) a common message that your Inner Critic harasses you with:

01

A CARTOON FIGURE THAT I FIND IMPOSSIBLE TO TAKE SERIOUS IS:

02

A COMMON MESSAGE FROM MY INNER CRITIC IS:

Great, in a moment you'll close your eyes and use your incredible imagination because you can: Imagine that your cartoon character is your Inner Critic. It starts telling you all the things it usually harasses you with BUT in the voice, mannerism, and style of your cartoon character. Really let it come to life in your imagination. Make it more and more ridiculous by modifying its voice, tone, pitch, and behavior until you notice you can't take it seriously anymore. Let Tweety lecture you. Or let Roadrunner say "merp merp!" when coming in and out of the picture to criticize you. You may notice a smile, a sigh, or some other form of physical response. We're looking for that physical response of relief.

JOURNAL

Now try to take the voice of the Inner Critic seriously again. What do you notice? It might be really hard to believe this voice now. Remember this as a tool to discharge any of its future attempts at putting you down.

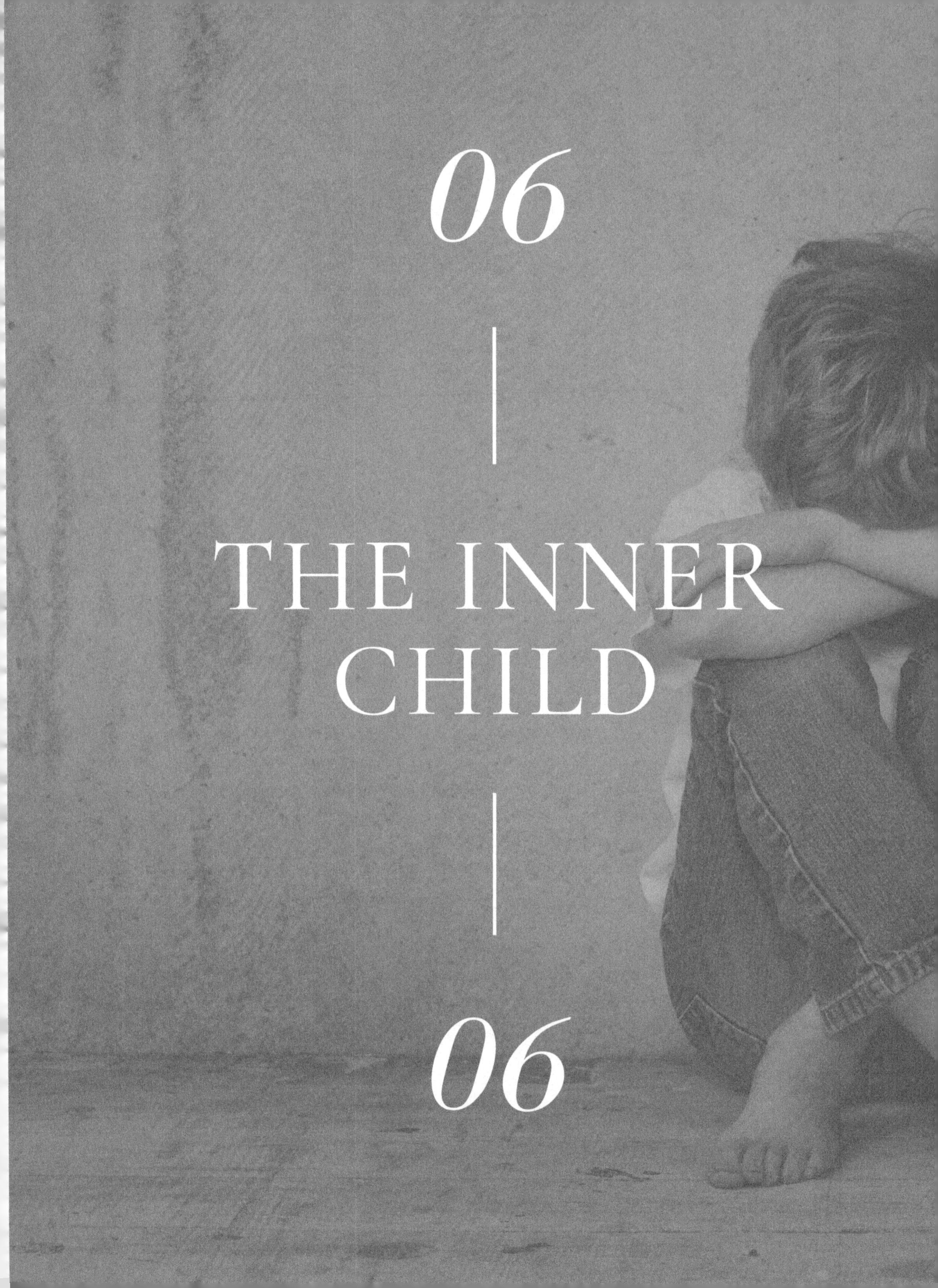

06

THE INNER CHILD

06

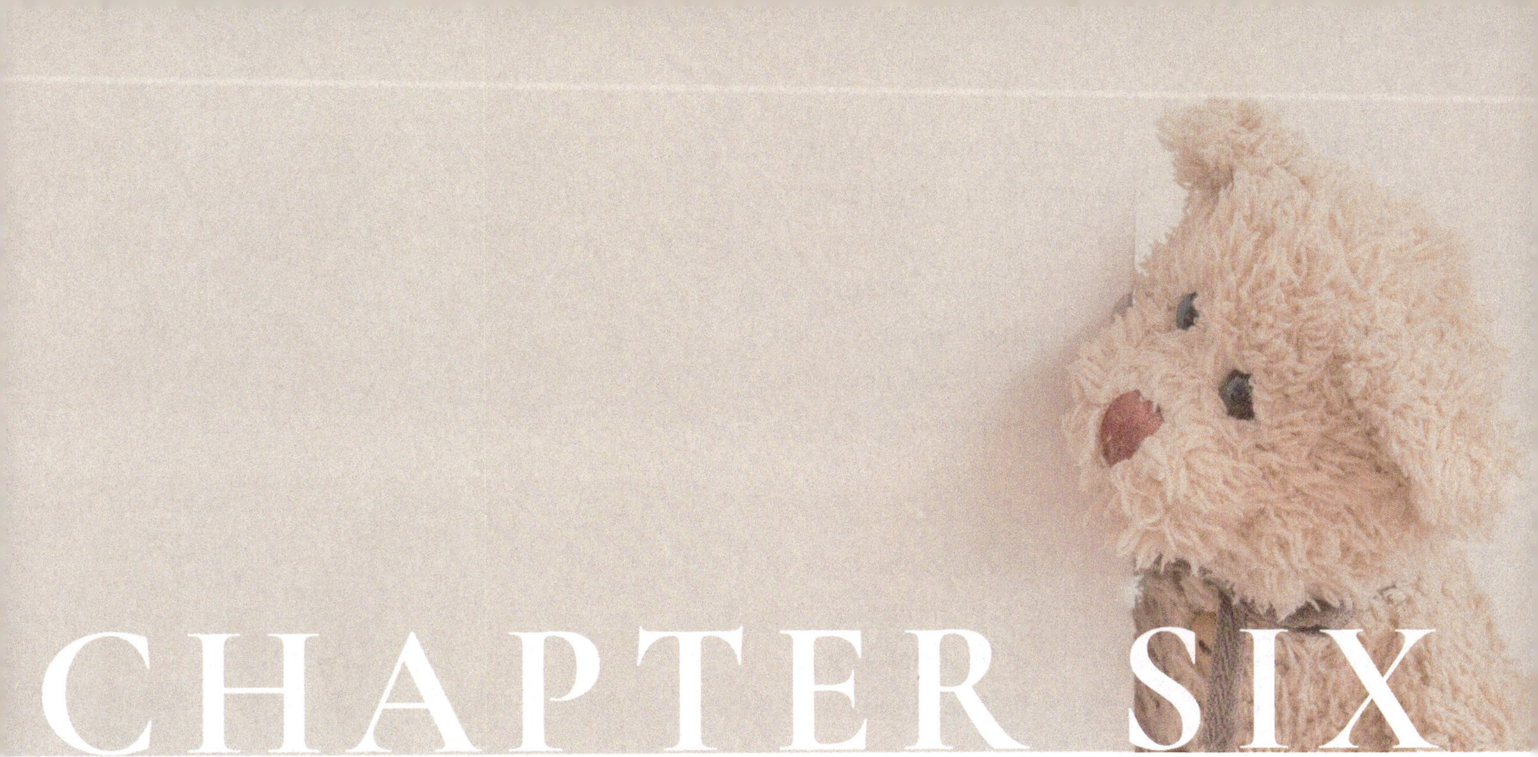

CHAPTER SIX

INTRODUCTION

Inner Child Work

06

Remember that our brains operate in theta brainwaves and we're little sponges until the age of 7? If it doesn't ring a bell, you can read up on it in Chapters 1 and 4. It's the reason why Inner Child Work is such an integral part of Shadow Work. We need to help our Inner Child through the pain, anguish, fear, and disempowering meanings they've given experiences in the past. Our Inner Child is stuck in the past and replays the same emotions over and over. Much like endless torture.

When I work with my clients, Shadow Work and Inner Child Work go hand in hand. We work to rescue the Inner Child from past pain and lead it back to safety and love. Unless we make our Inner Child feel safe with new perceptions, meanings, understanding, and resources, it will forever hold us back from experiences it deems unsafe and wants to protect itself from.

These kinds of childhood beliefs and patterns often have no logic. I often hear from clients, "The belief I notice is "XYZ" but I know it doesn't make sense!" It could be that we want the intimacy of a loving relationship, but at the same time, we push everyone away that gets too close. Objectively this doesn't make sense. But for the child within that has never grown past 3 years old it does make a lot of sense. S/he might be afraid of loss and carry an abandonment schema with a belief that says "intimacy is painful." S/he's afraid of being abandoned if s/he opens up and loves another dearly because when

Dad left during the divorce s/he made it mean that s/he wasn't worthy enough for him to stay.

Objectively, it doesn't make sense because as adults we know that's not what happened. Dad didn't leave because our Child Self was unworthy of love. But you aren't reasoning with an adult part, you are connecting to a child part.

That child part within never grew past the time of the trauma. It is stuck in the past, replaying the same pattern over and over in hopes of avoiding the same pain it felt when it first happened. It's a protection mechanism.

We don't consciously choose to do this. It is a shadow that lives in our subconscious. We need to bring the light of awareness to break the patterns, heal the Inner Child, and liberate it from its pain. What we see externally in our lives are only the manifestations of our Inner Child wounds. We create our external worlds based on the blueprint that is within us.

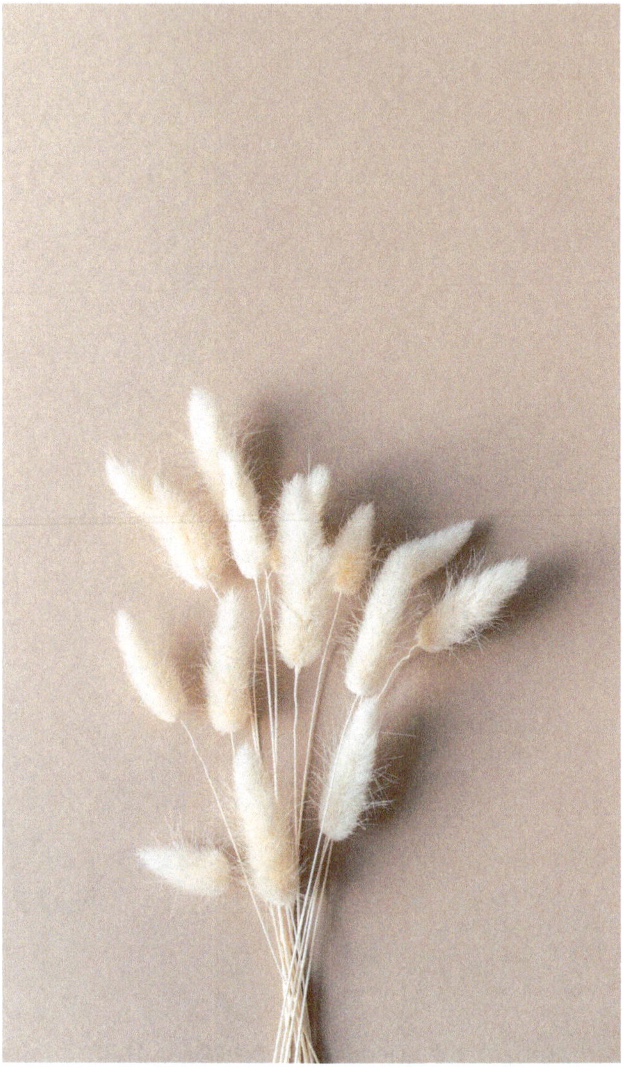

KEY POINTS TO REMEMBER

- *Children are in theta brainwave state until age 7, which means they receive the bulk of their programming or "conditioning" during this time.*
- *From age 7, this conditioning becomes part of the unconscious mind. It can be seen as a base programming that executes in the same kinds of situations.*
- *The adult will execute their lives based on the beliefs in the subconscious without consciously knowing why they do certain things.*

Journal PROMPTS

01 *What is your very first memory? Bring yourself back there and explain in detail, please.*

02 *List 3 of your favorite memories from your childhood. What made you feel did you feel in each of these memories? Use the Feeling Wheel if you need help clarifying the emotions.*

03 *Now look over those 3 memories – do they have something in common? Did they feel the same? Please share:*

Journal PROMPTS

04 *What is your worst memory? What did you feel? Why was it so challenging?*

Important: If this is a traumatic event please go only as far as you can without re-traumatizing yourself. Reach out to a professional if you need healing. I also offer Private Trauma Healing to help my clients, if you feel resonance.

05 *Which one of your needs went unmet in that moment? What did you really need? Please explore:*

Journal PROMPTS

06 *How did you have to change yourself in that moment in order to stay safe, loved, or provided for?*

07 *What did you have to believe about yourself to survive this challenging experience? "I'd have to believe that..."*

08 *What beliefs about yourself did you draw as conclusions from this experience? List them out below:*

Journal PROMPTS

Fully connect to your inner child now. Imagine that you are him/her in this moment. See through his/her eyes, feel your little body, and connect to your innocence. Let your inner child answer the following questions:

09 *How do you feel at home? What are your baseline feelings?*

10 *What emotion comes up often for you?*

11 *What is the narrative that accompanies this emotion? What do you tell yourself?*

Journal PROMPTS

12 *What is your tendency when you feel this emotion? What do you do?*

13 *What do you actually need and crave to feel safe, loved & accepted?*

14 *How can "adult-you" support you in receiving this? What do you need from them? Share freely without limitations below, "If I could ask for anything it would be..."*

INNER CHILD

Journal PROMPTS

15 *Who's love did you crave the most – your Mom's or your Dad's?*

16 *Who did you have to be to connect with this parent and receive love?*

17 *Who could you never be around this parent because this would have meant disconnection and loss of love?*

Section One

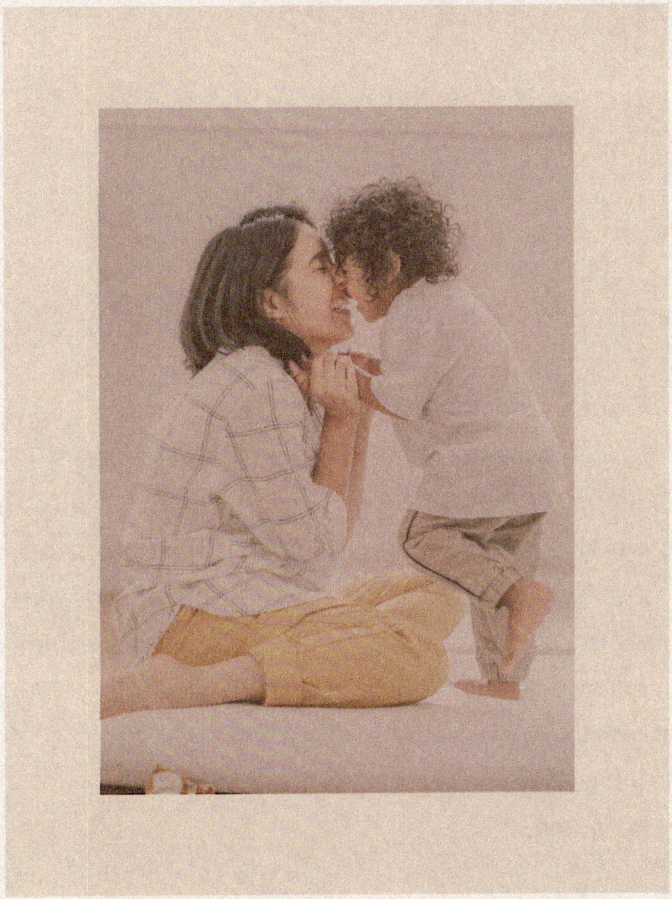

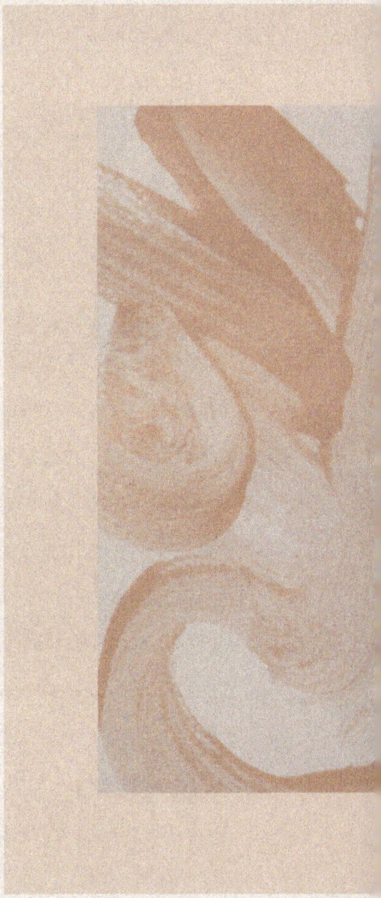

THE MOTHER WOUND

Healing The Relationship With Our Mother

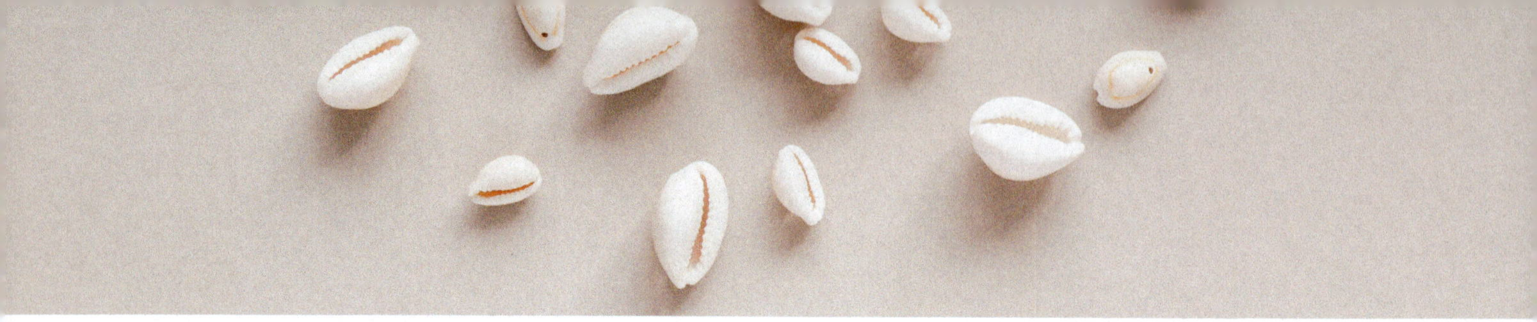

6.1 THE MOTHER WOUND

The largest predictor of human health and happiness isn't wealth or safety - it's the number of loving relationships we have. The first 3 months out of the womb are called the "4th trimester". Dr. Harvey Karp coined this term and explains that babies are born too soon. The babies' brain becomes too big in utero so we basically birth our babies prematurely. We should see our newborn babies as a fetus outside the womb.

Dr. Allan Schore, a leader in attachment theory, stresses that the basis of lifelong psychobiological well-being is established during the first 1000 days of our lives. He calls these first days "the origin of the early forming subjective implicit self." Neuroscience tells us that - to the brain - emotional pain and physical pain are the same. It can't differentiate between the two. Kelly McDaniel who wrote the book "Mother Hunger" explains that an infant in those early 2 years of life who is hungry or lonely feels pain, this would be literal physical pain if we trust the neuroscience.

"Where there isn't a close caregiver to relieve her, the pain intensifies. Her brain can't inform her body about why she's in pain. If maternal care is compromised during the first three years, this lack of nurturance is heartbreaking for a baby." Now think of what happens in our current society - women are forced to return to work way too soon from the point of view of the baby.

In the USA mothers are expected to leave their newborns when they are still in their 4th trimester. In other countries, there is a bit more support, but still, we get ripped away from the nurturance of our mothers prematurely. Children's brains double in size from birth until the age of 2 and we rely heavily on our mother's nervous system and nurturance to make sense of the world in this preverbal phase. McDaniel found through countless

hours of therapy we need 3 things from our mothers and if one of these isn't provided for we'll create strategies that - while they mean survival in the moment – harm us later on in life. These 3 things we all need from our mothers are nurturance, protection, and guidance.

Why am I telling you all this? Looking through the lens of these three needs can be truly enlightening to understand what we may have lacked in childhood. This helps us bring awareness and support to these parts of ourselves. I want to emphasize that this is not an exercise in blaming our mothers or making them wrong. We need to always remember that (unless you had an abusive mother) they did the best they could with what they had available based on what they were given. They are also only a product of their own conditioning and had their own struggles and challenges in life. I feel it's a common theme that we want to do better from generation to generation but we won't get it perfectly right either. And we don't need to. What is more important than unattainable perfection is that we showcase healthy repair skills, acknowledge our child's feelings, and are curious about their view of the world. Unless we condition our kids away from their inner truth they already know what's right for them. They have spot-on intuition. We can support them in finding the solutions and ways of living that really resonate with them. So, please don't judge yourself about how good a mother you are if you have children of your own. Remember, you also do the best you can in each moment with what you have available. Even if you think you could've done more. You couldn't. Please only look at this section from the perspective of your *own Inner Child*. The healing you do for yourself will be passed down through the generations, energetically and practically, no matter how old your children are now. Heal yourself and you'll heal the whole lineage.

And for the men: You too can have a mother wound to heal, it may just manifest slightly differently than it does for women. The aspect of guidance won't be as important because naturally, you will look towards male role models to learn from when you move into that phase of development.

Again, in this next chapter please focus on finding healing for yourself and keep the Shadow Work tips from Chapter 2 in mind as we progress.

IMPORTANT NOTE

Being raised by a single parent who met your needs, or growing up in a household with an atypical family structure that was generally healthy and loving, is not a cause of a mother or father wound. Mother and father wounds are caused by parents who were in your life but were neglectful or abusive on a level that left you unprotected, unsafe, and feeling as if you were unloved and too alone with your needs. But remember, sometimes we experience neglect despite the best efforts and full love of our parents. It's all about what we make situations mean internally as a child.

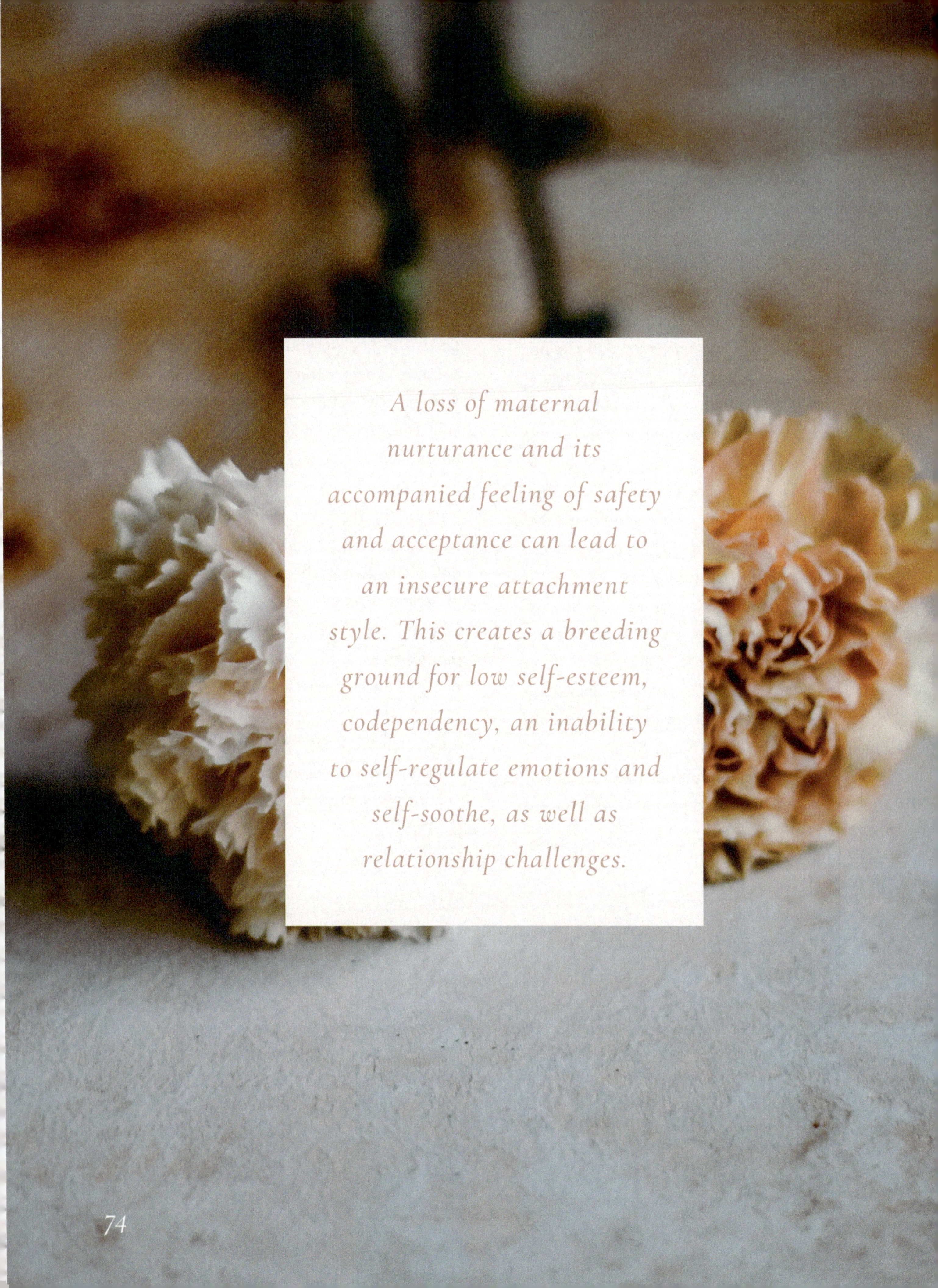

A loss of maternal nurturance and its accompanied feeling of safety and acceptance can lead to an insecure attachment style. This creates a breeding ground for low self-esteem, codependency, an inability to self-regulate emotions and self-soothe, as well as relationship challenges.

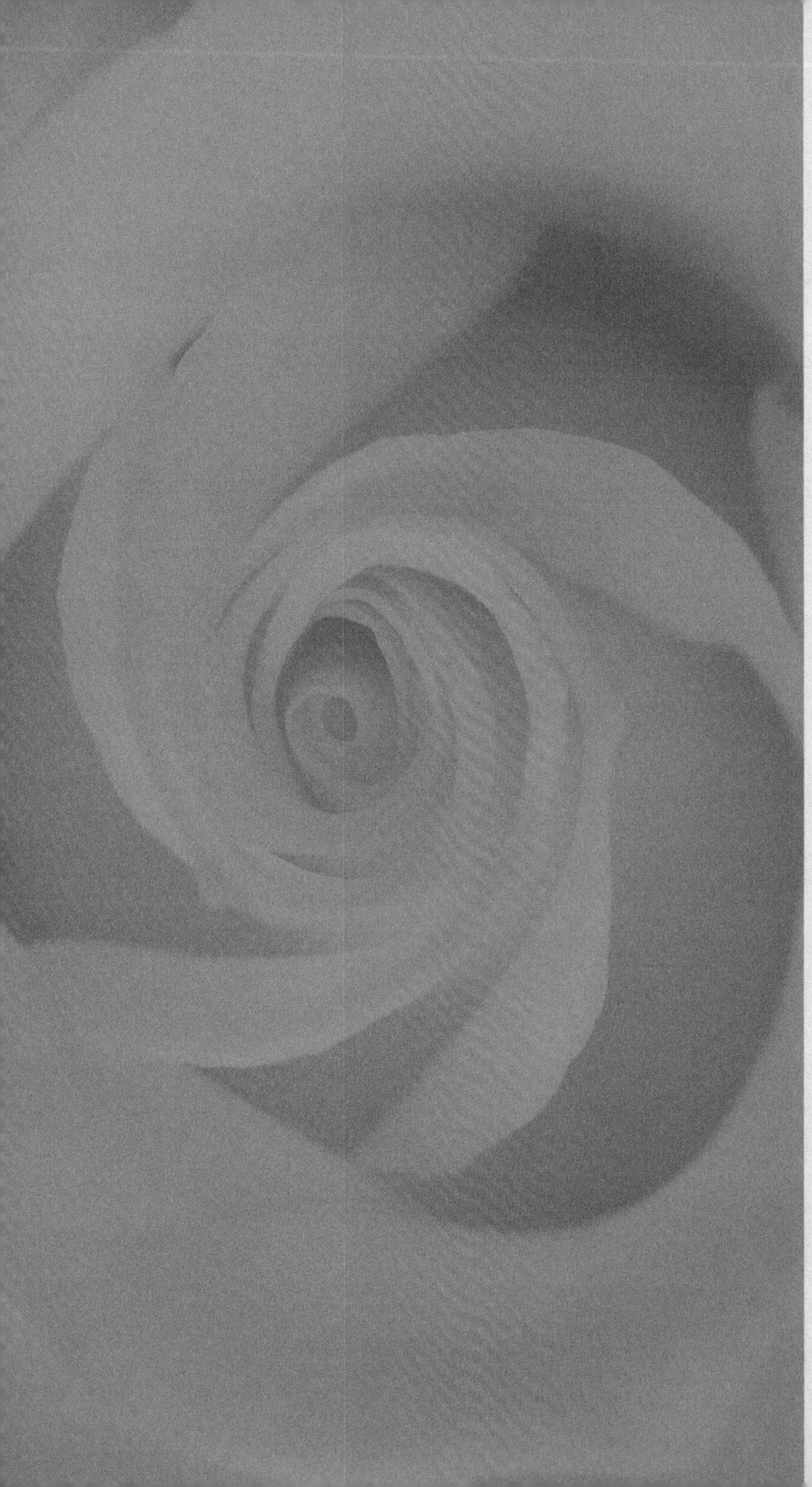

nurturance

Journal PROMPTS

01 *Was your mother emotionally available for you as a child? Explain, please.*

02 *Did you turn to your mother for comfort when things were difficult? Describe how that went and how it felt, please.*

03 *Who did you have to be to receive love and attunement (loving attention) from your mother? Explain, please.*

Journal PROMPTS

04 *Who could you never be around your mother? Being this way would've meant loss of attunement:*

05 *Did you feel like your mother could meet your needs? What did it feel like? What needs did and didn't get met? How did your mom react when you voiced needs:*

06 *How did my Mom deal with my emotions? Explain, please.*

Journal PROMPTS

07 *How do I deal with strong emotions now? What is my usual pattern? Explain, please.*

08 *How did I need to be met? How do I need to learn to meet myself now? Answer both.*

09 *If you had a magic wand – how did you wish your mother had nurtured you? Explore, please.*

Journal PROMPTS

10 *How would that motherly nurturance have felt in my body, mind, and spirit? Why? Please share below:*

11 *How can you, as your adult self, cater to these needs of your Inner Child now and make him/her feel nurtured? Brainstorm ideas for everyday life below:*

Replacing Lost Nurturance

When we didn't get the nurturance we needed in childhood we may experience we may find surrogates for the missing maternal love because we need to soothe ourselves. We may have been "good babies" because we didn't cry much but it may just mean that at some point we gave up hope that a caregiver would show up for our needs. As adults, we can give ourselves what our younger selves didn't get. Trying to find people who can give us the nurturance we need is helpful because it's a relational injury and can best be healed through nourishing relationships. Here are a few ideas for replacing lost nurturance.

- *Take hot baths or use soaking tubs*
- *Practice mindfulness and calming breath exercises*
- *Explore restorative Yin Yoga*
- *Try trauma-sensitive body work*
- *Ground in nature and try a gravity blanket*

NOTES

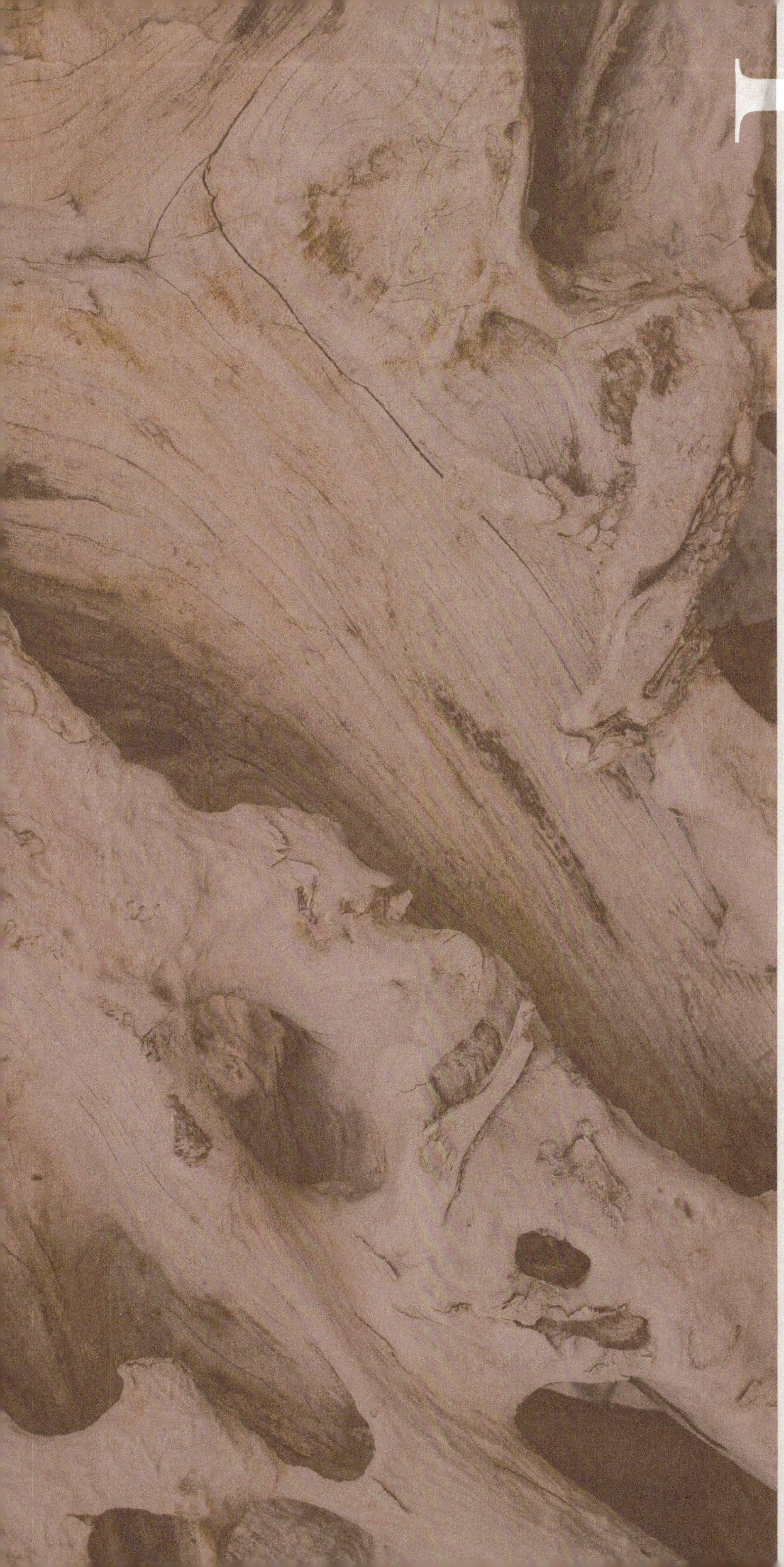

protection

Journal PROMPTS

01 *As a child, did you feel protected by your mother and safe around her? Why, why not?*

02 *Were there any situations where your mother may have failed to protect you (even though she might have done so if she had been aware)? Please share:*

03 *Did you turn to you mother if you needed safety or protection? How did that feel? Please explore below:*

Journal PROMPTS

04 *How did you create safety in childhood? What were your strategies? Do you still use them? Please, explain.*

05 *Did you feel you had to take on more responsibility than you could handle? Why, why not?*

06 *Did you feel like you had to take responsibility for mother's emotional or physical needs? Why, why not? How did that feel? Please, explain.*

Journal PROMPTS

07 *Did you feel like your mother should've protected you from someone or something and she didn't? Please, explain.*

08 *If you had a magic wand – how did you wish your mother had protected you? And how would that have felt? How would you be different now? Please, explain.*

09 *How can you, as your adult self, cater to these protection needs of your Inner Child now? Brainstorm ideas for everyday life below:*

Replacing Lost Protection

When we didn't get the protection we needed from our mothers in childhood we may have constant low-grade anxiety, panic, sleep disorders, and a sense of being younger than our age. We may have even taken on a sense that we need to protect our mother. Here are a few ideas on how you can replace lost protection.

- *Find your right balance with scary and stressful media*
- *Set clear boundaries around touch*
- *Use your nervous system regulating exercises*
- *Try trauma-sensitive body work*
- *Ground in nature and try a gravity blanket*

NOTES

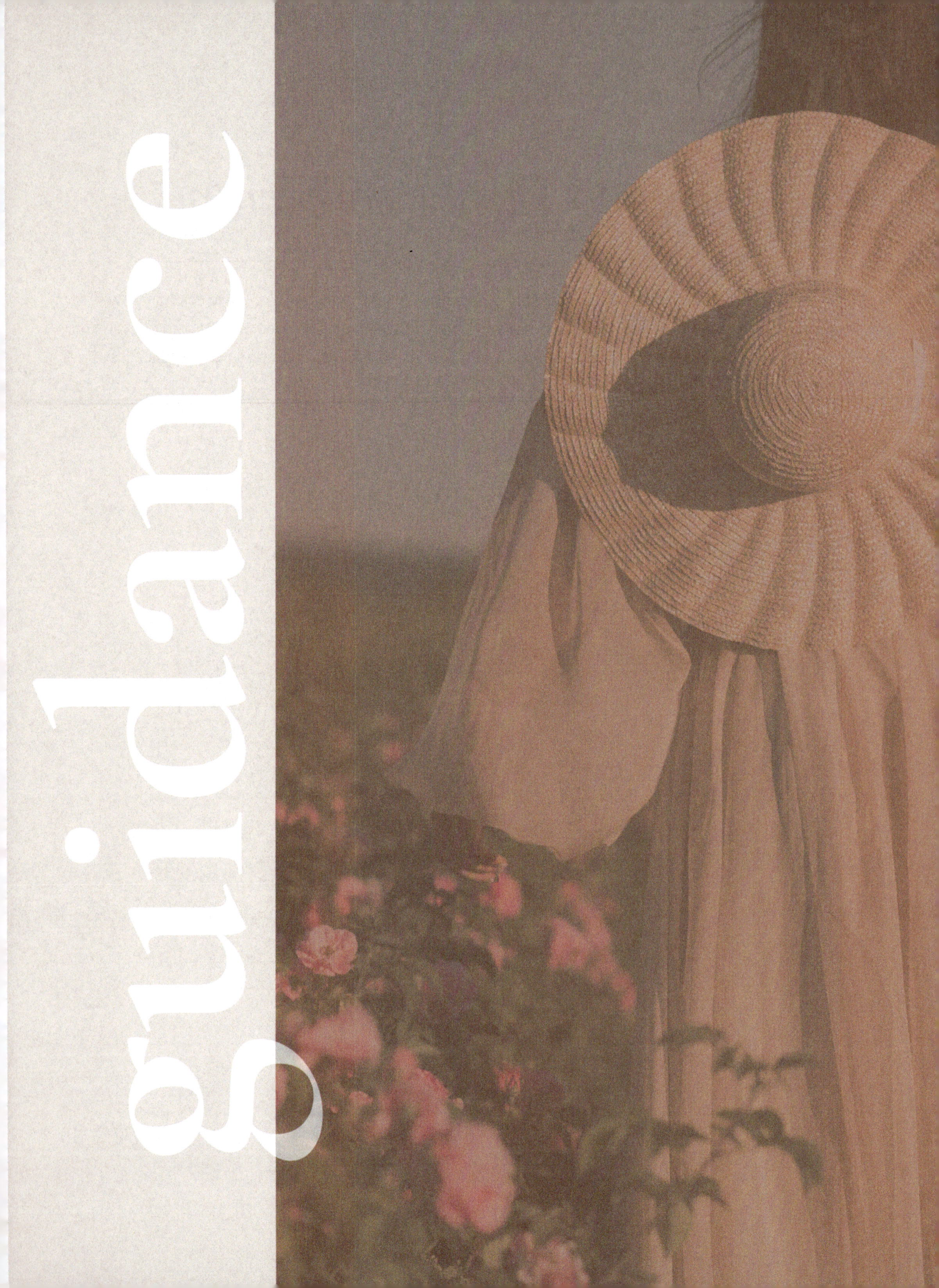
guidance

Journal PROMPTS

01 *Do you feel like you can confide in your mother and receive guidance and support? Note: As women, we never outgrow the need for healthy maternal guidance. Gentlemen, this is relevant for you as well and we'll go deeper into fatherly guidance in the next Chapter.*

02 *Did this evolve over time by working on yourself or has this connection always been there? Why, why not. Explain, please.*

03 *Was your mother able to empathize with your needs and problems so you felt truly understood, seen, and heard? Please explain.*

Journal PROMPTS

04 *How has your mother's guidance usually felt? Supportive or intrusive? Could/can you receive it or did/do you reject it? Please explain.*

05 *Did your mother ever give you unsolicited guidance and how did this feel? How did your body feel in those moment? What was your impulse and reaction? Explain, please.*

06 *If you had a magic wand – how did you wish your mother had guided you?*

Journal PROMPTS

07 *How would it have felt or would it feel if your mother gave you guidance in a way that feels supportive and appropriate to you? How would you feel different? How would your relationship be different?*

08 *How can you, as your adult self, cater to these needs of your Inner Child now? Brainstorm ideas for boundaries and positive relating in everyday life:*

Replacing Lost Guidance

When we didn't get the guidance we needed in childhood we may rely on ourselves rather than getting help. We grew up too soon and may be the "independent one". We may long for role models and inspiration, someone to look up to and learn from. We are also vulnerable to getting exploited and having others misuse power over us. Whether we have had a mother who gave unsolicited guidance, guidance that felt wrong, or didn't show enough interest in our world, it can leave a wound. And this may still persist to this day and can keep feeling painful to us. Here are a few ideas for replacing lost guidance.

- ✓ *Set clear boundaries about guidance with your mother*
- ✓ *Find a coach or mentor*
- ✓ *Explore learning something that interests you*
- ✓ *Build your intuition and inner guidance*
- ✓ *Ground in nature and let her whisper to you*

NOTES

food

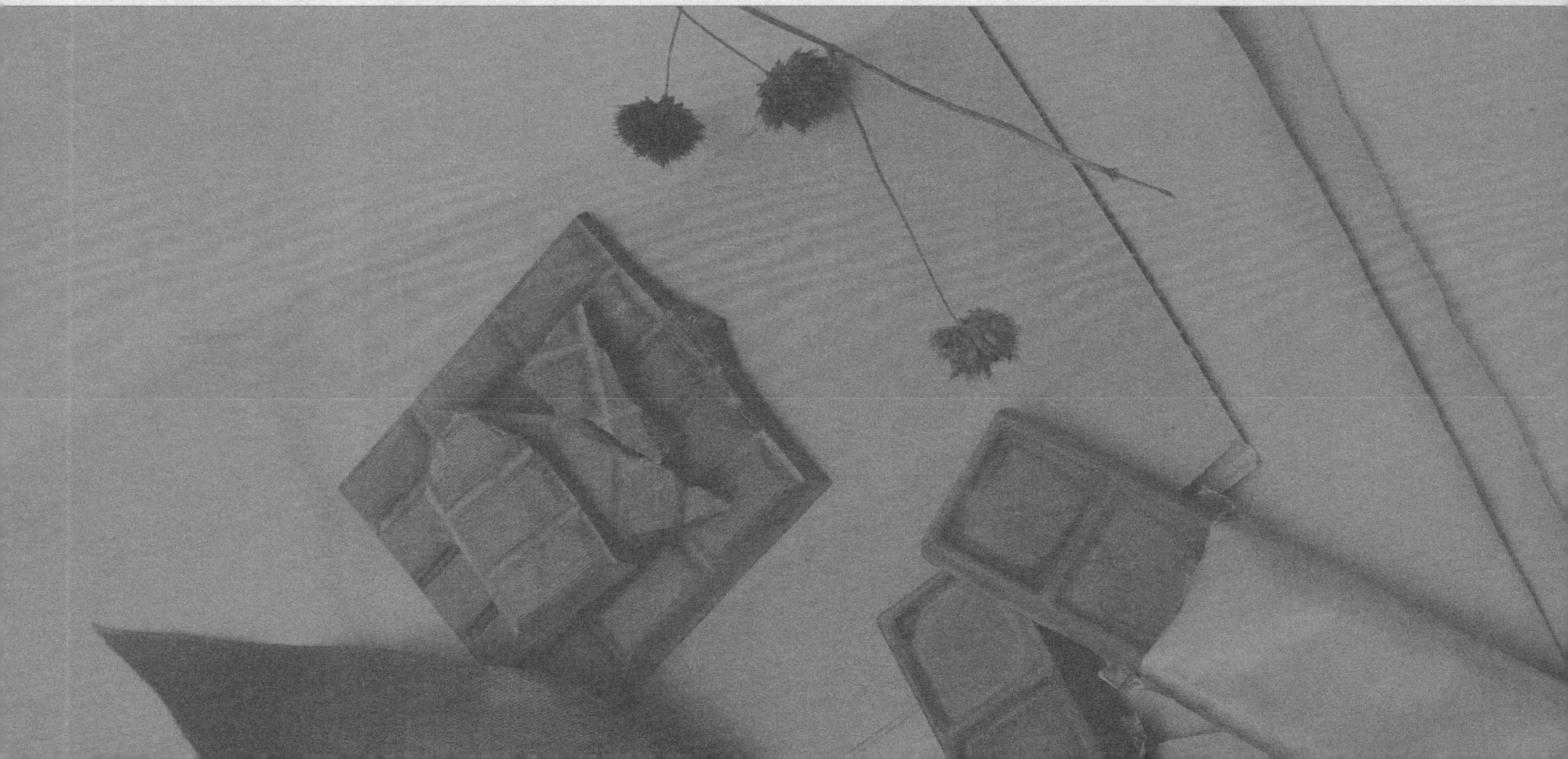

Journal PROMPTS

01 *Were you ever encouraged to eat as a child? Was it around certain foods or in general? How did this feel?*

02 *Were you ever deprived of food or didn't get your favorite foods? Please explain.*

03 *Was eating a social thing or did everyone eat at different times? How did this feel?*

Journal PROMPTS

04 *Did you binge or sneak food as a child or teenager? Explain why and how.*

05 *Did you deprive yourself of food or restrict food in adult years? How so?*

06 *As an adult, do you know when you're hungry? What are the signs for you?*

Journal PROMPTS

07 *What is your favorite food? Why? What emotions do you connect with it?*

08 *Please describe three feelings you have about food or mealtime.*

09 *Apply those three words to intimacy. What do you notice?*

Journal PROMPTS

10 *What is your relationship with food like? Do you eat when you're hungry, emotional, or bored? Do you forget to eat? Do you crave it and feel guilty after? Are you very functional about it? Do you eat the same things repeatedly? Do you eat a lot of sweet foods? Do you (over)exercise to "balance out" food intake? Explore your behaviors and emotions below:*

11 *Has it always been this way? When did this start? Did one or both of your parents eat in a similar way? Explore where your relationship with food comes from below:*

12 *What is the pattern that you are starting to notice now? Do you overeat or undereat? Do you not allow yourself food? Do you numb yourself with food? Do you feel triggered when you're too full or too empty? Do binge and/or restrict? Journal below:*

Journal PROMPTS

13 *Well done. In what other areas of your life is the same pattern that you have with food presenting itself? Is it a theme that shows up in your romantic life, business or career, finances, friendships, or health? How so? Please explain.*

14 *What do you make it mean about yourself that this pattern is playing out?*

15 *What do you feel you deserve or don't deserve based on this belief?*

Journal PROMPTS

16 *In what ways has this belief about yourself affected your results in relationships/work/finances/health? List out each one.*

17 *What strategies do you have to keep affirming this belief as true?*

18 *What strategy have you adopted to mask the pain of this belief?*

Journal PROMPTS

19 *In which aspects of life do you not feel nurtured?*

20 *If you had a magic wand – how would you want to feel different?*

21 *What would you really love to be able to do/be/have that you don't allow yourself based on this belief?*

Section Two

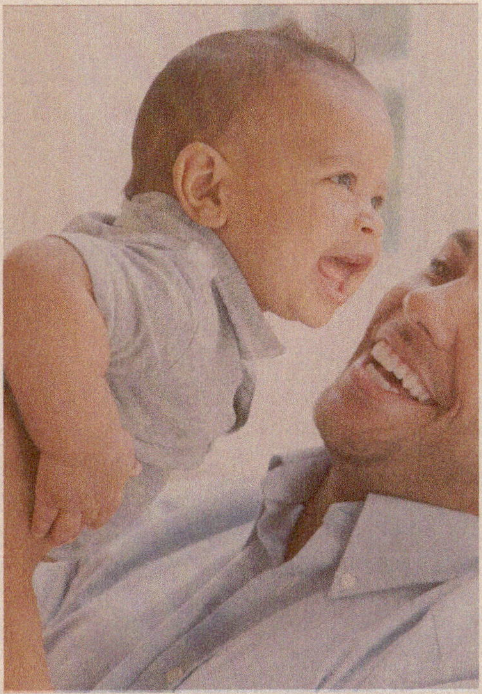

THE FATHER WOUND

Healing The Relationship With Our Father

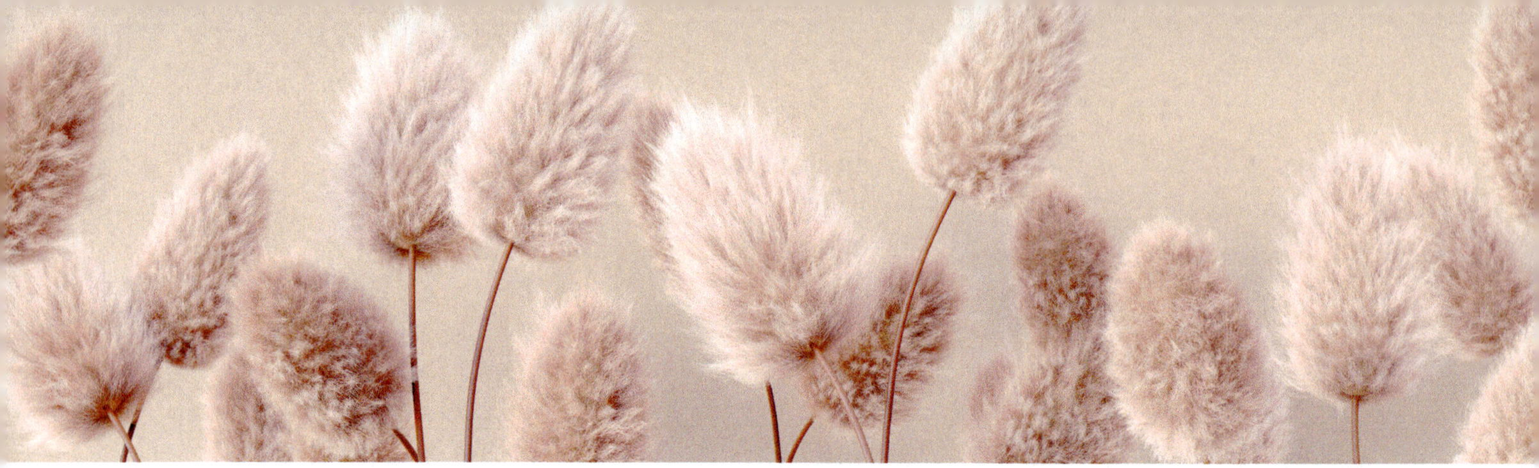

6.2 THE FATHER WOUND

The father wound and the mother wound can be similar in their causes – typically, the result of absenteeism, emotional neglect, abuse, or an unattuned parent or caregiver. But the impact of each wound can be very different based on our different cultural models for what we expect to get from our mother versus our father.

Our father's role is oftentimes associated with physical protection and guidance on how and who to be in this world. The feminine qualities a mother offers and the masculine qualities a father offers can be viewed as distinctly different in purpose. The power of a woman lies in bridging the spiritual and physical realm to bring life onto earth. She creates the child from her own cells and life force energy over many months. She creates life. In her full power, the feminine can bring wisdom to her children and man about the spiritual nature of the world. A man on the other hand has strength in the physical realm. He is physically stronger and is naturally designed to navigate and master the physical experience.

A father's role is to teach and prepare the child to survive and succeed in the world. Often fathers are able to teach the harder lessons of life better than a mother can because of her nurturing instincts. He'll be able to bear a child hurting itself under the umbrella of learning more than a mother could. Fathers have an integral role to teach us how to navigate and succeed in this world so that we are physically safe and know how to thrive independently.

When we miss our father's protection, have felt their lack of guidance, or approval of our actions in the world it can leave deep wounds in our sense of self. In this section, we will have a deeper look at the relationship with our father and how it has influenced who we are today.

FATHER WOUND

Journal PROMPTS

01 *What is your favorite memory of your father? How did you feel in that memory? Why? Describe it here.*

02 *What is your worst memory of your father? Why? How did you feel? What happened? Describe it, please.*

Journal PROMPTS

03 *What was your relationship with your father like in childhood? How did you two relate? How did you feel towards him? Take a moment to describe it.*

04 *What is your relationship like now? Describe it in your own words.*

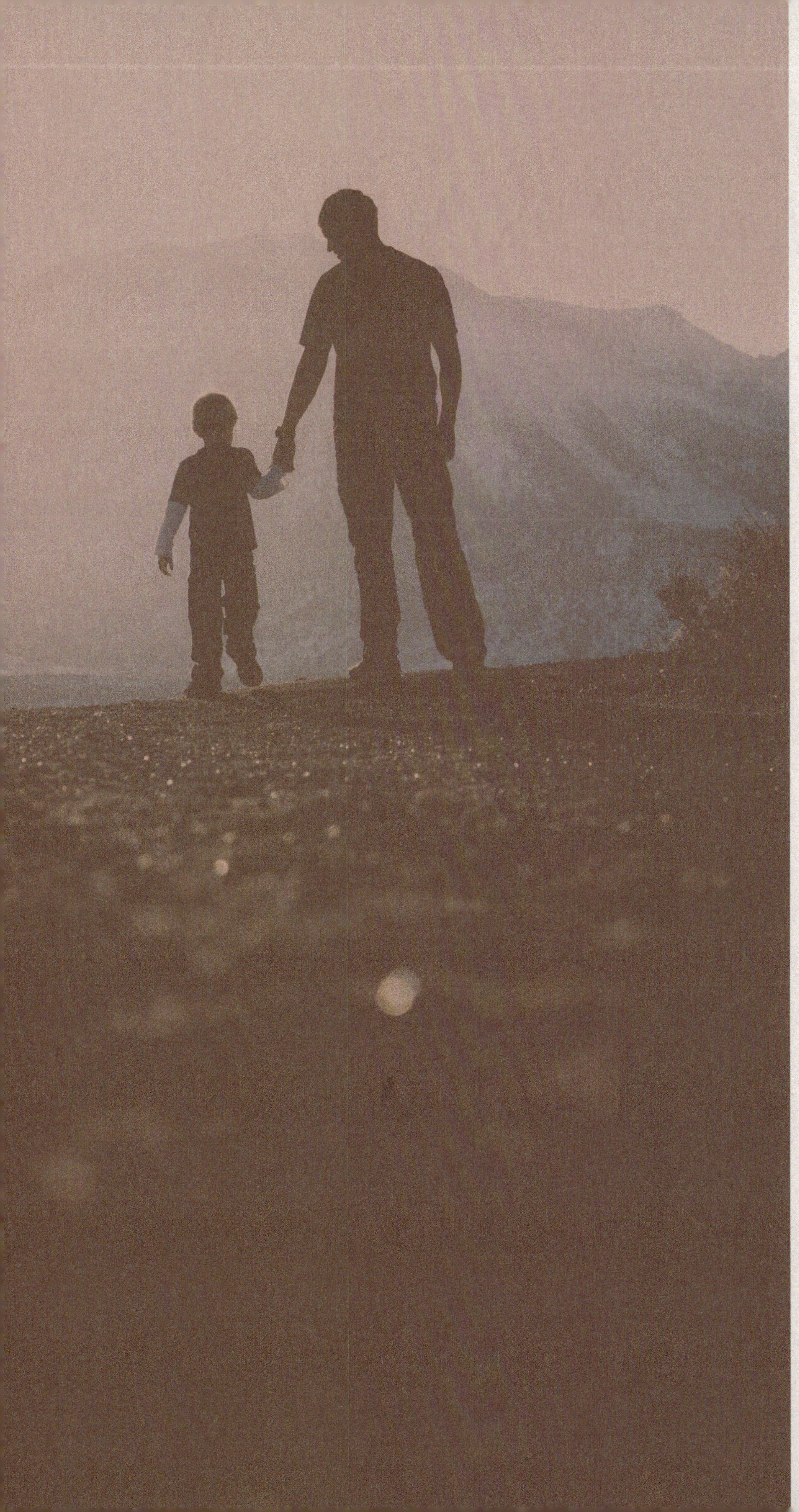

attunement

Journal PROMPTS

01 *Was your father emotionally available for you as a child? How so?*

02 *Did you turn to your father for support when things were difficult? Why or why not?*

03 *Who did you have to be to receive approval from your father? Explain, please.*

Journal PROMPTS

04 *Who could you never be around your father? Being this way would've meant loss of attunement:*

05 *Did you feel like you need to prove yourself to your father? How so?*

06 *Did you feel like your father could meet your needs? What did it feel like? What was missing for you?*

Journal PROMPTS

07 *How did Dad deal with your emotions? What was his usual response? What did he direct you to do? Please, explain.*

08 *How do you deal with strong emotions now?*

09 *How did you long to be met as a child? And how can you meet myself now to cater to these needs?*

Journal PROMPTS

10 *Did you feel your father was emotionally available? Why or why not?*

11 *How has this impacted you in your life? Please explain.*

12 *How is this being reflected in your relationships throughout life? Take a moment to look at the overarching patterns and explain below:*

Journal PROMPTS

13 *If you had a magic wand – how did you wish your father had attuned to you in childhood? Be specific.*

14 *How would that have felt emotionally, physically, and mentally?*

15 *How can you, as your adult-self, cater to this need of your Inner Child now? Brainstorm ideas for everyday life:*

Replacing Lost Attunement

the way we experience the loss of paternal attunement can be quite different depending on whether we are male or female. A loss of paternal attunement can lead little girls to keep choosing emotionally unavailable partners that too can't give us what we need. For little boys, this loss can lead to low confidence and overcompensation. As adults, we are able to cater to our needs and choose the right people that support us and enrich our lives. Here are a few ideas but please brainstorm your own:

- ✓ *Discover your attachment style*
- ✓ *Weed out people who reflect the loss pattern*
- ✓ *Use your nervous system regulating exercises*
- ✓ *Try trauma-sensitive body work*
- ✓ *Work on your self-worth*

NOTES

protection

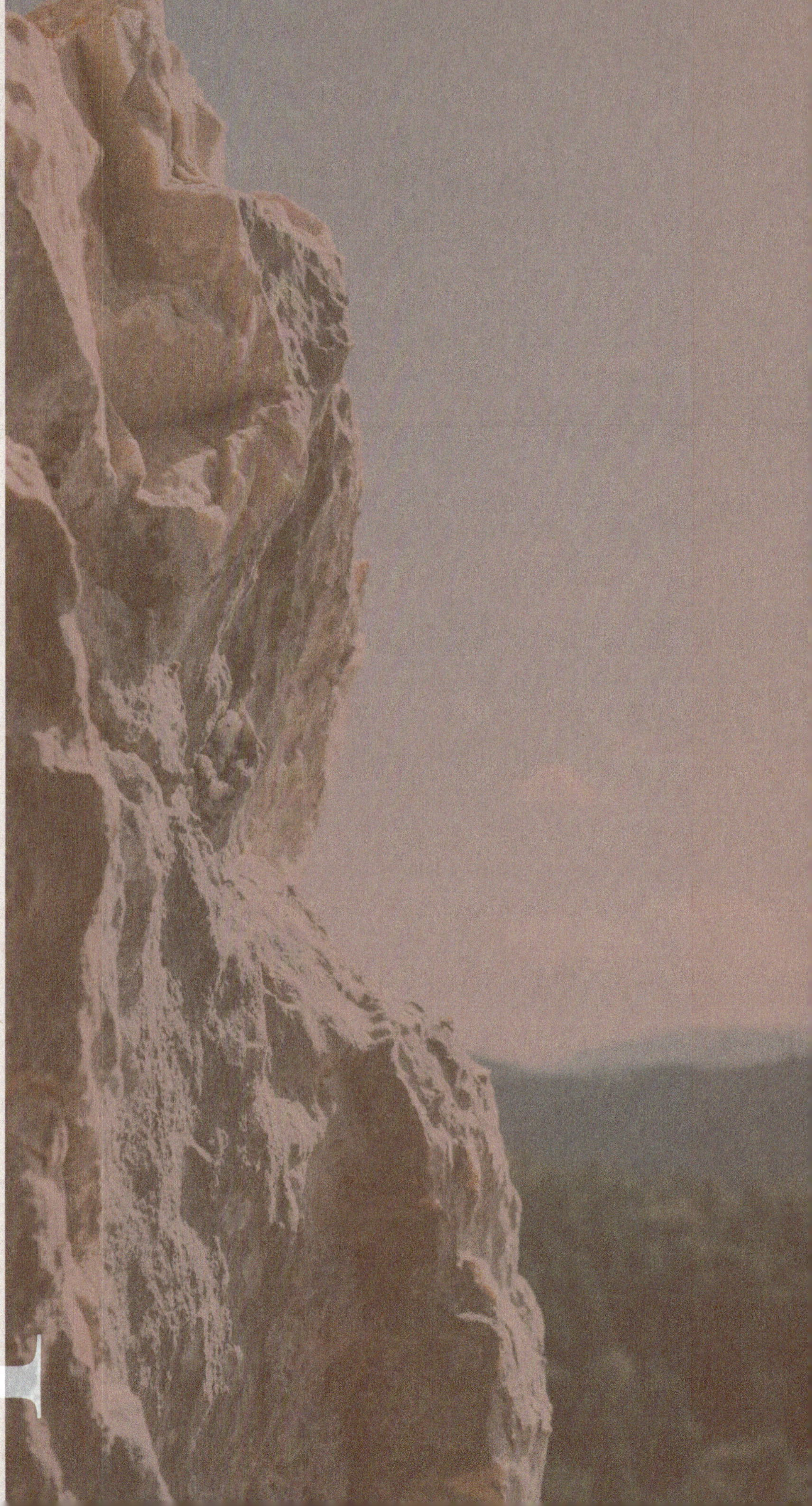

Journal PROMPTS

01 *As a child, did you feel protected by and safe with your father? Please explain.*

02 *Were there any situations where your father failed to protect you (even though they might have done so if they had been aware)? How so? How did that feel? Please explain.*

03 *Did you turn to your father for protection as a child? Why or why not?*

Journal PROMPTS

04 *Did you feel like your father should've protected you from someone or something and he didn't? How so? How did that feel? Please explain.*

05 *If you had a magic wand – how did you wish your father had protected to you in childhood?*

06 *How would that have felt? Be specific.*

07 *How can you, as your adult-self, cater to this need of your inner child now? Brainstorm ideas for everyday life here:*

Replacing Lost Protection

When we didn't get the protection we needed from our father in childhood it can lead to similar expressions as the loss of maternal protection. We may have constant low-grade anxiety, panic, sleep disorders, and a sense of needing a thick wall to keep people out. We may have even taken on a sense that we need to protect our father. Here are a few ideas on how you can replace lost protection.

- ✓ *Find your right balance with scary & stressful movies*
- ✓ *Set clear boundaries around touch*
- ✓ *Use your nervous system regulating exercises*
- ✓ *Try trauma-sensitive body work*
- ✓ *Explore martial arts, cardio kickboxing or boxing*

NOTES

guidance

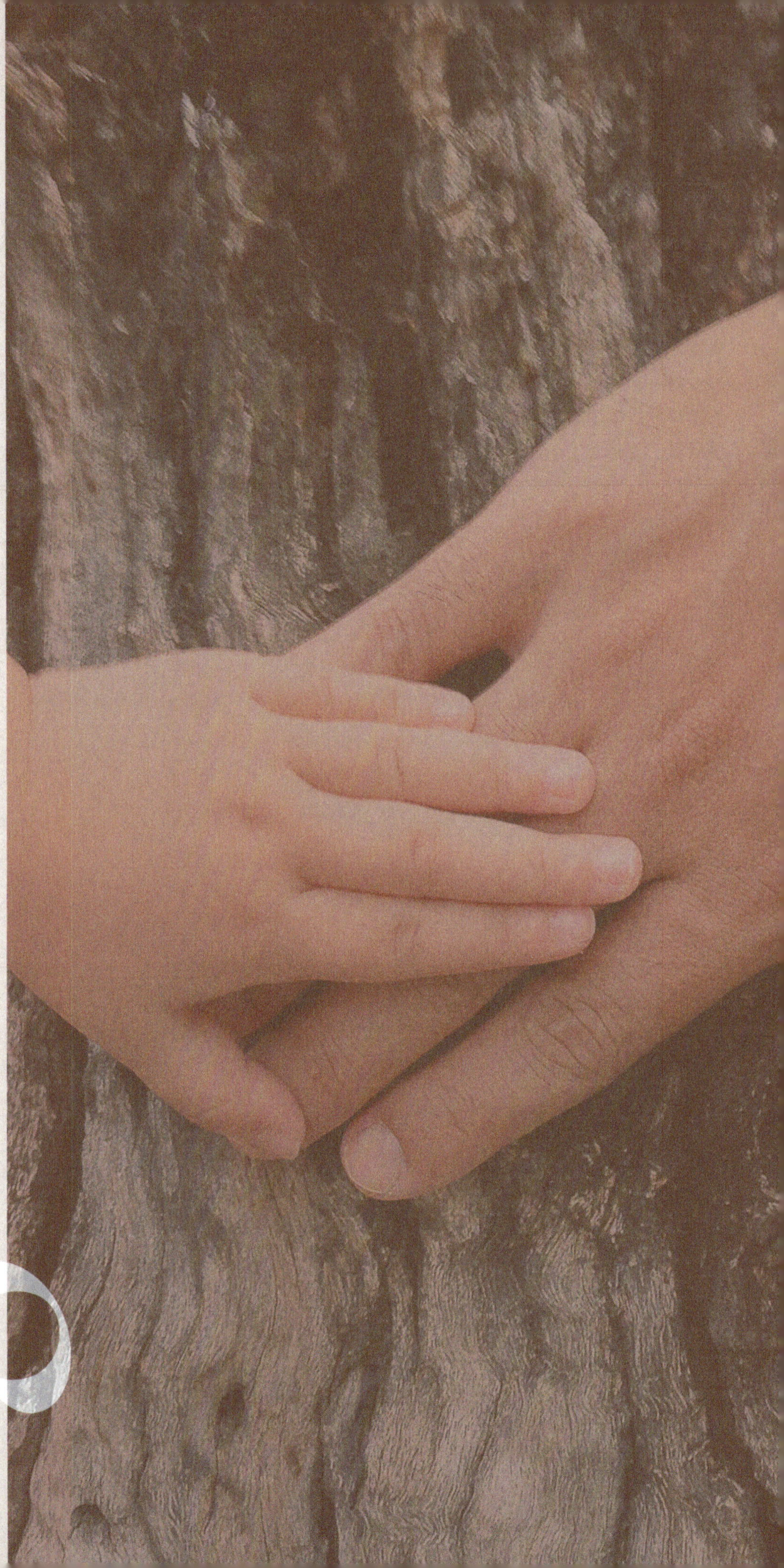

Journal PROMPTS

01 *Do you feel like you can confide in your father and receive guidance? Note: This is especially important for men when they come of age and are looking for a male role model to teach them about manhood. Describe, please.*

02 *Did this evolve over time by working on yourself or has this connection always been there? Please explain.*

03 *In which ways did your father teach you about the world and your place in it? How did that feel? Please describe it.*

Journal PROMPTS

04 *Did you feel like this was what you needed or were you missing an aspect of guidance? Was the delivery helpful and did it work for you? Could you receive it? Please describe.*

05 *How has your father's guidance usually felt – emotionally, in your body and mind? Please explain.*

06 *Did your father ever give you unsolicited guidance and how did this feel?*

Journal PROMPTS

07 *Did your father ever give you unattuned guidance that seemed "wrong" for you and how did this feel?*

08 *What need for guidance went unfulfilled by your father in childhood and beyond?*

09 *If you had a magic wand – how do you wish your father had guided you into adulthood? Please describe.*

Journal PROMPTS

10 *How would that have felt – on an emotional but also a physical level? Explain, please.*

11 *How can you, as your adult-self, cater to this need of your Inner Child now? Brainstorm ideas for everyday life now:*

Replacing Lost Guidance

When we didn't get the guidance we needed in childhood we may rely on ourselves rather than getting help. Similar to the loss of maternal guidance, we may have grown up too soon, be very responsible, and self-sufficient, or could be seen as the "independent one". We may long for role models and inspiration, someone to look up to and learn from. Someone who can make us feel safe in this world. We are also vulnerable to getting exploited and having others misuse power over us. When we had a father who couldn't properly prepare us for the world or tried too hard and imprinted limiting beliefs, we can heal now. Here are a few ideas for replacing lost guidance.

- ✓ *Find an excellent coach or mentor*
- ✓ *Learn about finances, investing, and wealth*
- ✓ *Explore learning something new that interests you*
- ✓ *Build your intuition and inner guidance*
- ✓ *Watch shows that teach you about the world*

NOTES

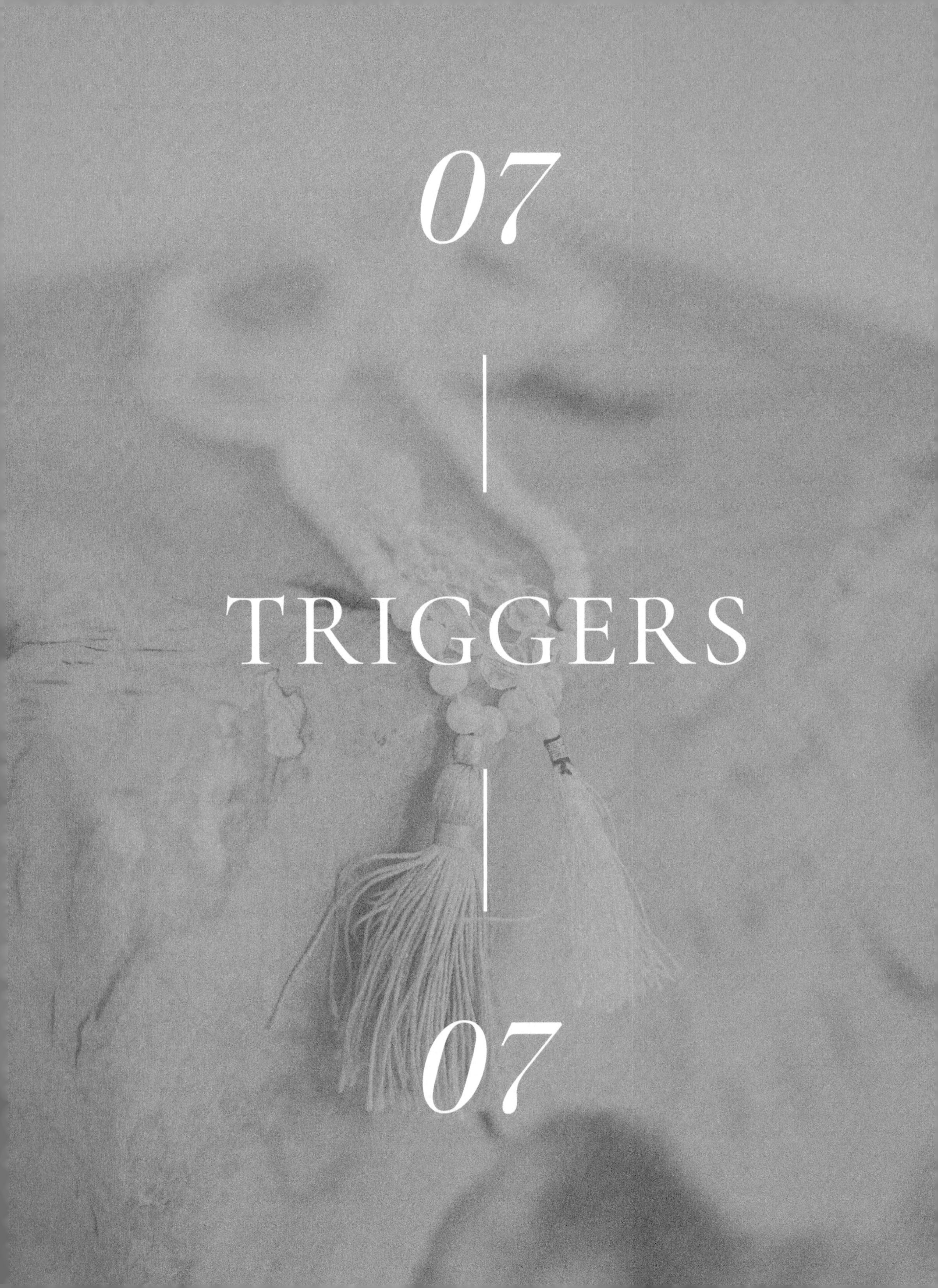

07

TRIGGERS

07

MODULE 7

Transcending Triggers

By definition, we aren't conscious of our own unconscious aspects. We need to search for the truth through questioning, contemplation, and attention to our own behaviors, thoughts, and reactions. These reactions are often called triggers. Triggers are reactions to experiences that remind us of previous trauma.

Triggers illuminate our wounds just like a stage light sets the focus on a performer. We can recognize a trigger as a strong emotional reaction to a situation that doesn't warrant the intensity of our response. They seem to rise up out of nowhere and can be unleashed explosively toward others or even ourselves.

We default into a trauma response and usually have 1 of 4 strategies: fight, flight, freeze, or fawn. When we're triggered we feel such strong physical sensations that make it feel impossible to react any other way. Language often gives us clues about the truth: re-action. It is not a new action that we are coming up with at the time of a trigger. It is a *re*-action, so an action that has happened before and we are only repeating it. We are re-actioning the past. Re-enacting a moment in childhood that has imprinted itself in our subconscious.

We had an experience in our past that resembles what is happening now. Since we haven't healed this specific wound it still controls our present and will influence our future unless we release it. This is the gift of Shadow Work. We can free ourselves from the certain future that resembles the same patterns and results of the past.

NOTES

When we are courageous enough to look at our shadows, even though it will be uncomfortable and confronting, we can release the tight grip that these unconscious patterns and beliefs have on our lives. They've made our lives *predictable* because we've relived the same patterns and allowed them to play out again and again. A belief or childhood wound is like a program running in our subconscious that will get us the same results without fail. Once we're fed up with being stuck in the same patterns and getting the same results, we finally find a resource like the book you are reading right now that can help us disclose our truth.

Triggers can be blessings that shine a bright light on unconscious patterns that usually hide in the darkness of our Shadow Self. It is a sacred situation, that allows us to see the wound and become curious about what shadow aspect is being mirrored back at us. Shadow Work through triggers can feel like a reactive process because we need to *wait* until we get triggered so that we can become conscious of our wounds.

NOTES

Remember that the whole world around us is a reflection of what is inside of us. If a person or situation triggers us it is a message *for* us. It is an act of service from the universe to help us see what is *inside* of us that is still unresolved. Once we heal these wounded parts of us we can free ourselves, our minds, our energy, and recreate our worlds.

I applaud you for your courage to gaze at your own shadows and let them transform in the light of awareness. You are liberating your inner self and with it, reinventing your life. Curiosity is paramount to understanding yourself and what need has gone unmet in the past.

Triggers are a gift! They can help you make huge leaps in self-awareness and boost your Shadow Work progress. Triggers are always rooted in childhood themes, wounds, trauma, and unconscious programming.

When we can understand what the root cause of the trigger is we can give our Inner Child what it actually needs and free ourselves from these old coping strategies. On the next pages, you'll find tools that can help you with transforming your triggers.

WORKSHEET

Transforming Triggers

What is the trigger?

What is the current sensation, emotion, or energy in your body? Say it in a sentence, i.e. "I'm so angry my husband didn't clean the dishes again."

What is my first impulse?

What is the first re-action that follows the trigger? i.e. "I want to confront him and scream at him" (fight response)

What is underneath?

Your trigger is the coping strategy that has kept you safe. What do you or your Inner Child *really* need right now? What underlying need are you actually trying to meet? i.e. "be seen and heard in my needs so I can feel valued"

What do I make it mean?

How am I interpreting this situation? What do I make it mean about myself, the world, and my place in it? What's the story? i.e. "he doesn't care about my needs. My needs don't matter. I'm not seen. I'm not loved."

How can I reframe this?

Remember you are interpreting the world through your own filters based on your experiences. Ask yourself: Is my meaning objective truth? What else could it mean? i.e. "maybe he didn't feel well"

My new response is:

How could you respond not react (re-enact the past) instead? i.e. "I'll communicate calmly, set boundaries, hold him accountable"

WORKSHEET

Triggers as Mirrors

What is the trigger?

What is the current sensation, emotion, or energy in your body? Say it in a sentence, i.e. "My son says "no" to all of my requests. It's so hard to get him to do anything."

What is my first impulse?

What is the first re-action that follows the trigger? What do you feel and think? i.e. "I'm frustrated! He should just do what I tell him to, I'm not asking for much!"

What is the mirror?

What could this situation or person be reflecting back to you? How did you act in the same situation as a child? i.e. "When I was a child I just did what I was told and what was expected of me. It's not that hard!"

What part was disowned?

Describe what part of you never got to behave in this way and judges this situation or person. i.e. "When I was young I had to do as I was told. I couldn't say "no" just because. It made me feel trapped, and I found it frustrating. "

How did I want to feel?

How did your Inner Child really want to feel? What is it maybe even jealous of? i.e. "I wish I could've felt carefree as a child so I could explore, be light and free. Not carry so much responsibility."

My new response is:

If there were no limitations or consequences, how can you give yourself permission to live this feeling now? i.e. "I'll take less responsibility and allow myself to be carefree."

TRIGGERS

Journaling

REALIZATIONS

Inner Child Rescue

01 What is the trigger?

What situation triggered me and why?

02 What does it mean?

What does this mean about me, the world, and my place in it?

03 What do I feel?

What emotion surfaces as I feel this trigger?

04 What's underneath?

How is my reaction protecting me from feeling this: [write down feeling]

05 Where do I feel it?

Where does this sensation sit in my body? How does it feel? Give it a color, shape, density.

06 Is there a person?

Is this emotion connected to a person? Who comes to my mind first?

07 Hand it back

Pull this energy out of your body and hand it back to the linked person or to source energy.

08 Inner child rescue

What would I do for a child that feels this way? How would I want to help them?

09 Transformation

How does my Inner Child respond to my support? How do they feel now?

10 New role

Allow the child to drop the old role and choose a new role in your inner world. The new role is:

INNER CHILD RESCUE

Journaling

REALIZATIONS

Transcending Triggers

STEP BY STEP

1) What is the trigger & its meaning?

What situation triggered you, how did you react, and what did you make it mean? i.e. husband didn't do dishes, I feel angry & like my needs don't matter

2) Has a boundary been crossed?

i.e. Yes, we agreed he would do the dishes each evening

3) What do I need from the other person?

i.e. I need to feel like he values my needs and I can trust him to keep his word

4) What do I need from myself and how can I give it?

i.e. I need to prove to myself that I am valuable and that my needs matter. I will make sure that there is accountability so I can feel safe and valued.

5) What is my new boundary?

What is a new boundary you want to set or a new agreement that you want to make with someone?

6) How can I communicate my needs and boundaries?

Try the conscious language formula on the next page. What is a fitting situation to bring it up where we can all be calm and open? Good communication goes both ways.

Conscious Language

"I" language encourages communication without assigning blame. Often we think we are using "I" language but we are not. For instance, "I hate it when you leave your dishes on the bench" is not helpful "I" language. Although the statement starts with "I" it can still come across as accusatory and may result in the other person disengaging from the conversation. An "I" statement that opens up solutions might look like this: "I noticed you didn't clean the dishes last night. I feel angry because I make it mean that my needs don't matter and I'm not valued. It would really help me if the dishes could be cleaned in the evening." Give it a try!

I NOTICE

I FEEL

BECAUSE

WHAT I NEED IS

Apology Cheatsheet

Often we yearn for an apology to be able to move on and forgive. But we may never receive the apology, understanding, or remorse we need from the person. That's why we need to build our own inner sovereignty and hold ourselves in safety. In order to transcend old patterns and evolve our consciousness through relationships we need to be able to discern a *real* apology from a fake one. The fake ones keep us stuck in disempowering relationships with friends, partners, and family. Sincere apologies soothe our nervous system and help us in creating safety within and without.

WHAT'S NOT AN APOLOGY:

- ✗ **An excuse:** sounds like "I'm sorry I snapped at you but you're just so stubborn."
- ✗ **A denial of your experience**: sounds like "I'm sorry you feel this way" or "You're just too sensitive." The last one also adds insult to injury as if your experience happened in a vacuum that they weren't a part of.
- ✗ **Manipulation**: sounds like "I'm sorry I'm late, you know how unorganized I am." This is an act of trying to get your forgiveness without having earned it.

WHAT IS AN APOLOGY:

- ✓ A **real apology** consist of two parts:
- ✓ 1. **Recognition** of the pain caused
- ✓ 2. **Repair efforts** to soothe pain
- ✓ Sounds like: "I'm sorry I didn't let you know I was going to be late and that you were so worried. Next time, I'll text you on time so you can relax."

08

REPARENTING

08

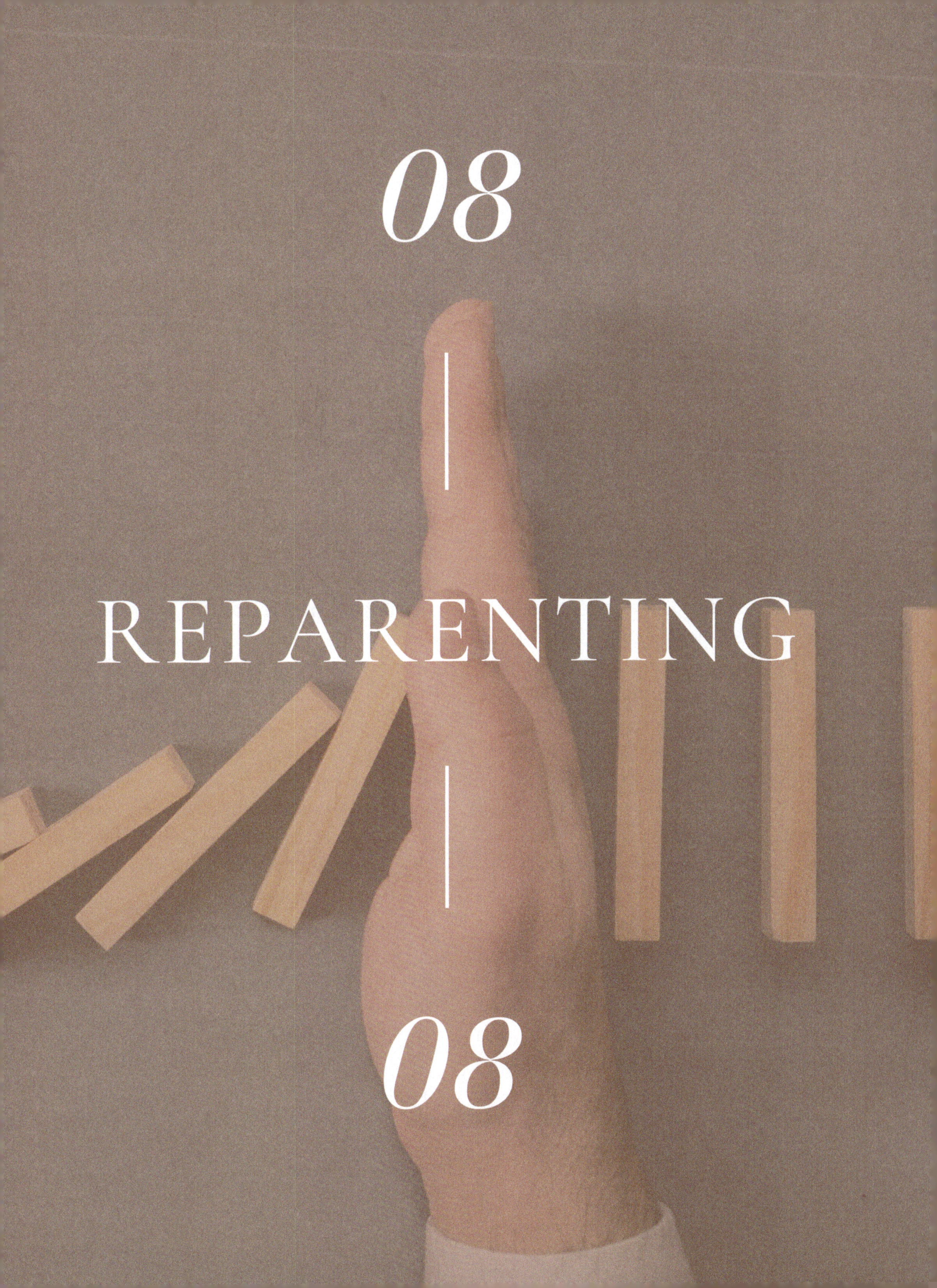

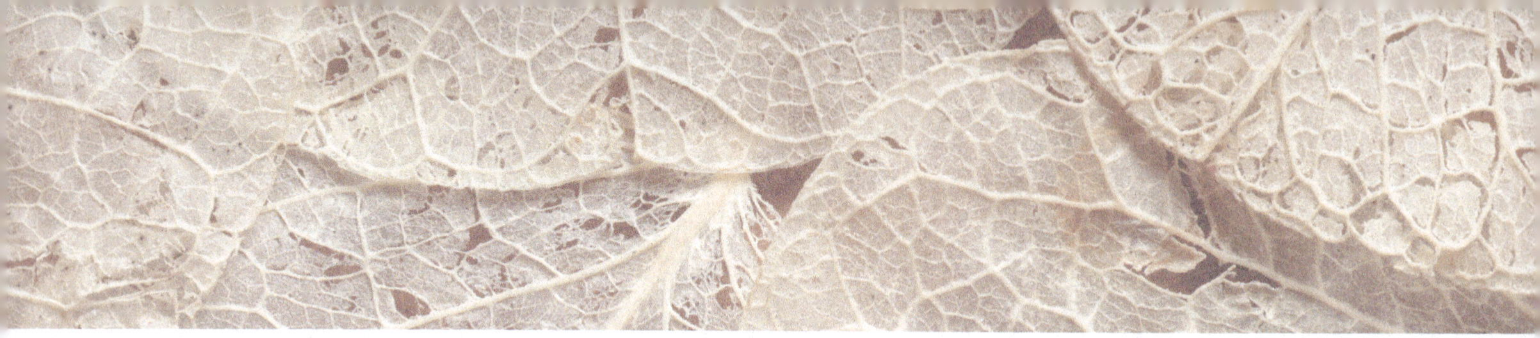

08

INTRODUCTION

Reparenting

Going through this book you've likely discovered quite a few beliefs, emotions, unmet needs, and maybe even trauma that you have carried all your life. Your Inner Child can't age past those moments of traumatic events. It has stored the beliefs that were created in the past and keeps running them just like a program keeps running on a computer. But we can delete or change them.

Let me explain to you how this works by giving you an example. Imagine you're 3 years old, playing with your toys. You've been content but now you feel like you need your Mom's attention for attunement. Your Mom is on the phone and her attention is elsewhere. She can't attend to you and she's out of attunement with you – she's busy and focuses her attention on other things. As an adult, you will look at this situation and think, "Okay, I'll just wait until she's done talking on the phone and is available. No big deal." For an infant, these logical functions of rationalizing and temperance aren't available.

Feelings, especially those of loneliness or abandonment, can be so intense that they are felt like physical pain. Remember, that neuroscience tells us that – to the brain – emotional pain and physical pain are the same. I've had clients that have formed lasting beliefs from similar situations in childhood. They seem harmless and would go completely unnoticed. But an impression of "I'm not important" or "Unless I'm loud my needs won't get met" imprinted with emotional intensity will become a belief that keeps playing out over and over until we allow this part of ourselves to find peace and return to truth and wholeness.

Remember what Leonardo DiCaprio's character says about an idea in the movie "Inception"? He asks, "*What is the most resilient parasite? A bacteria? A virus? An intestinal worm? An idea. Resilient. Highly contagious. Once an idea has taken hold of the brain it's almost impossible to eradicate.*"

When parents can't show up for us the way we need them to, we do not stop loving our parents – we stop loving ourselves.

These ideas that take hold of our minds are like parasites that keep draining our energies. We keep living out the same false interpretations of reality and begin to believe that we are less than lovable. But these ideas and subjective interpretations aren't the truth. They are only one interpretation of an objective reality as we've seen in the NLP Model.

Knowing this, we can reparent our Inner Child and soothe our minds. We can detach from the parasitic mechanisms in our minds that syphon off our energy and reclaim our power. We do this understanding that the Shadow Self was never evil, to begin with. It is only hidden. It is those experiences that were too painful to relive and re-feel so we pushed them into a dark corner of our psyche so we can keep functioning in our daily lives. Now we know though that the pain doesn't have to keep us captive. We can break free by returning to an inner space of self-love and self-acceptance. But we can't bypass our awareness and choice. We need to know *why* we decided to keep ourselves locked into this pattern and we need to make the choice to stop it. Yes, we are *that* powerful.

We were born knowing, connected to a higher wisdom, and with the innate power to create worlds from the infinite imagination of our minds. Now we get to reclaim ourselves. We get to say "no" to what doesn't feel right to us.

We get to stand up for our Inner Child that felt hurt, lost, alone, violated, and rejected. As the adult Self, we get to say "I got you" to our Inner Child and create a barrier of protection so that they can feel safe, loved, and worthy. With awareness, we are now able to reparent our Inner Child and cater to all the needs it felt deprived of.

NOTES

OVERVIEW

Reparenting Trifecta

We can't go back and change our childhood. So as adults, we need to become the parent that our Inner Child always needed. We need to give ourselves today what we craved in childhood but didn't receive. We need to protect ourselves from the same painful experiences and actively work on creating a trusting relationship with our own Inner Child.

01 NEEDS

02 BOUNDARIES

03 STANDARDS

EXPLANATIONS

01

NEEDS: In the previous chapters we've gained new insights about our childhood experiences. We now know that unmet needs leave wounds that crave healing and that we will keep creating the same experiences so that we can become aware of them, reframe their meaning, and take new actions.

02

BOUNDARIES: A boundary is a definite line where your responsibility ends and another's begin. It stops you from doing for others what they should do for themselves. A boundary also prevents you from rescuing someone from the consequences of their own destructive actions which they need to experience in order to grow. It can be confronting to set boundaries in the moment but in the long-term, you will create a membrane that protects you and teaches others how to treat you.

03

STANDARDS: A standard is a minimum requirement or quality that needs to be present to entertain another in any sort of relationship.

OVERVIEW

Reparenting the Self

The most important relationship we have in life is the relationship with ourselves. Being able to trust ourselves to do what we promise ourselves to do builds our confidence over time.

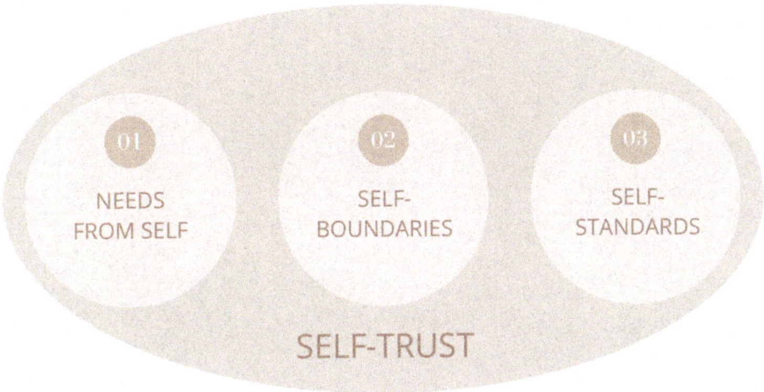

BUILDING SELF-TRUST

01

How can you cater to your own needs? Do you even know your own needs? Do you respect them, inquire about them, and make sure that you take good care of yourself? You can't expect anyone else to look after you if you're not willing to do it for yourself because as you now know life is a mirror. You have to show yourself you are worthy to attract people who respect your boundaries and needs.

02

Do you enforce your boundaries? Also to yourself? Knowing your own boundaries is only one aspect of healing – the other is enforcing the boundaries even when it feels confrontational or uncomfortable. If you decided you will no longer be self-destructive in certain aspects, remember that small child within – they really need you to show up for them! They are hurting and need protecting.

03

Make sure you set new standards on how you allow yourself to be treated – by you! We can forget that we are often the most destructive force in our own lives and the way we speak to ourselves is so harsh that we would never dare to do that to others. How can you increase the standards on how you hold and treat yourself?

OVERVIEW

Benefits of Boundaries

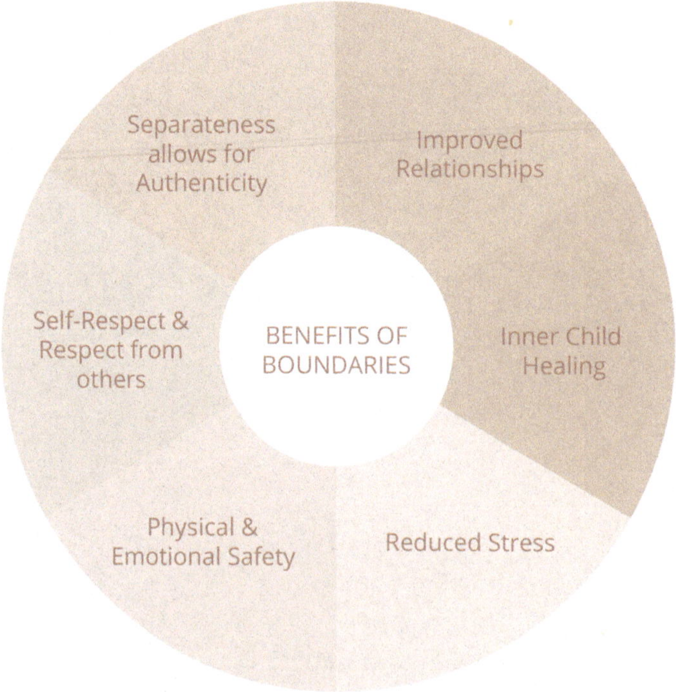

Clear boundaries are a gift that you give yourself. At first, it can feel uncomfortable to be exposed to other people's emotional reactions to your boundaries but you have to remember this: either you keep abandoning yourself to please others or you keep yourself safe and let other people figure out their own emotions. It's a simple choice: Do you choose yourself? Or do you choose them? And still another perspective: You are actually depriving others of the triggers they need in order to grow. You could be that mirror for them to see a pattern that is unconscious to them and they could heal.

NOTES

BOUNDARIES

Journaling

REALIZATIONS

WORKSHEET

Monitoring Boundaries

S

Situation

In what situation did I let my boundaries be crossed? Why?

D

Dissociation

What was the trigger and how did my body react in the moment?

T

Thoughts

What thoughts were going through my mind in the moment?

A

Afterward

How do I feel about myself now? What does my inner voice say?

WORKSHEET

Needs and Boundaries

01 *What safety needs did I discover went unmet in my childhood?*

MY NEW BOUNDARIES ARE:

02 *What attunement needs went unmet in my childhood?*

MY NEW BOUNDARIES ARE:

WORKSHEET

Needs and Boundaries

03 *What protection needs went unmet in my childhood?*

MY NEW BOUNDARIES ARE:

04 *What guidance needs went unmet in my childhood?*

MY NEW BOUNDARIES ARE:

Friend Boundaries

HOW YOU WANT TO FEEL:

I want to feel like I can trust my friends. I need to know that I can open up to them and that what I tell them will be received with empathy and care. I don't want to be interrupted or told what to do unless I specifically ask for guidance because I realize I don't feel heard if someone only listens to fix me. I need my friends to be punctual or to tell me on time if they will be late so that I don't feel like my time investment is disrespected. I need to know that I can trust their word and rely on them when I need them even if it may be a bit of an inconvenience for them. I like to feel like it's an open and honest space where we can share our needs and respect each other's capacity to cater to them from a place of compassion. I will also make sure that I respect limitations to their capacity but will not abandon myself or my needs. I'll make sure to check compatibility before I let people too close to me.

3 BOUNDARIES

01 *Be on time or let me know as soon as you know what arrival time I can expect*

02 *If I find out that I'm being lied to or deceived I will cut contact*

03 *I won't share deeply personal things until I know that I can trust this friend with delicate topics*

STANDARDS

1. *Have similar life values*
2. *Being able to have enriching, positive conversations*
3. *Emotional maturity*

etc.

WORKSHEET

Self Boundaries

HOW YOU WANT TO FEEL:

3 BOUNDARIES

01

02

03

STANDARDS

WORKSHEET

Family Boundaries

HOW YOU WANT TO FEEL:

3 BOUNDARIES

01

02

03

STANDARDS

WORKSHEET

Friend Boundaries

HOW YOU WANT TO FEEL:

3 BOUNDARIES

01

02

03

STANDARDS

WORKSHEET

Work Boundaries

HOW YOU WANT TO FEEL:

3 BOUNDARIES

01

02

03

STANDARDS

WORKSHEET

Partner Boundaries

HOW YOU WANT TO FEEL:

3 BOUNDARIES

01

02

03

STANDARDS

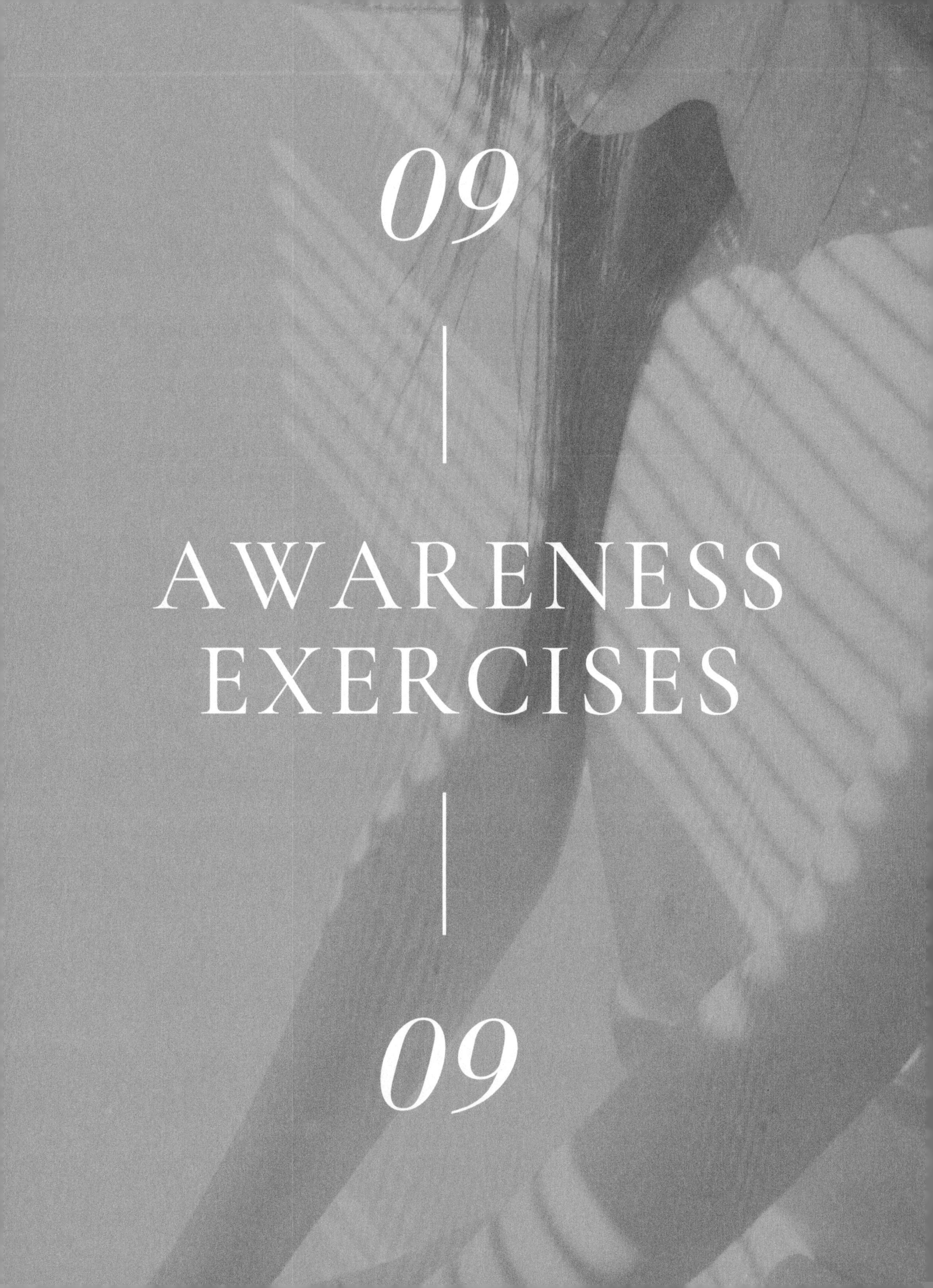

09

AWARENESS EXERCISES

09

ONGOING PRACTICES

Awareness Exercises

This is the part where we pull all of the insights that you've gained over the last chapters together. It serves as a summary and steady practice for you so that you can keep growing through your inner work. Shadow Work is an ongoing process. At any given moment in time, we can only access those unconscious parts that are alive and ripe for us to heal. The inner work of healing and awakening to our True Self is often described as an upward spiral because we may revisit a theme or pattern a few times before we can fully shift it and let it drop out of our experience. If you continuously attract a pattern there is still something that you're not seeing as it hides in the Shadow Self. Remember, the external world is only a reflection of your inner world. You attract what you need to experience in order to be guided back into wholeness and a higher expression of consciousness. But some things we just can't see as we do the work alone – some patterns are so deeply buried and hidden that we need a skilled Shadow Work Guide or therapist to help us. If you're looking for further support please feel free to check out my offerings. But for now, let's dive into this last chapter together and tie all the awarenesses together for continued growth.

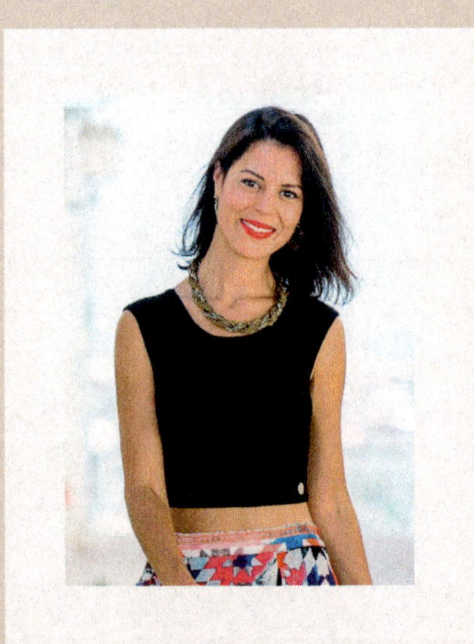

Shadow Work is a life-long devotion to your soul's growth and expansion of consciousness. As long as we ignore what is hidden we are imbalanced in our expression and easy to manipulate. I cheer you on to grow in your power and find liberation.

xx Sharon

AWARENESS

Schemas & Themes

In the first chapter, you've learned about 18 schemas that can play out as themes in our life. Let's revisit what they were and note them down here. Start with the one that feels strongest down to the weakest.

01

SCHEMA / THEME

02

SCHEMA / THEME

03

SCHEMA / THEME

04

SCHEMA / THEME

AWARENESS

Unmet Childhood Needs

What are the three biggest needs that went unmet in your childhood? Revisit all your notes and the journaling you've done in this book and summarize it here to have a clear overview.

01

02

03

JOURNAL

01

02

03

PRACTICE

Shifting Triggers

Q *What is one trigger that I uncovered?*

Q *What is the childhood wound that created this trigger?*

Q *What is my underlying need that requires attention so that I no longer get triggered?*

HOW IT USED TO PLAY OUT	HOW I'M HANDLING IT NOW

PRACTICE

Achieving Goals

01 *What is my conscious goal?*

02 *What is a repeating unconscious pattern or belief that gets in the way of achieving my goals?*

03 *How does it manifest itself to sabotage me?*

MY SOLUTION IS

PRACTICE

Integrating Your Identities

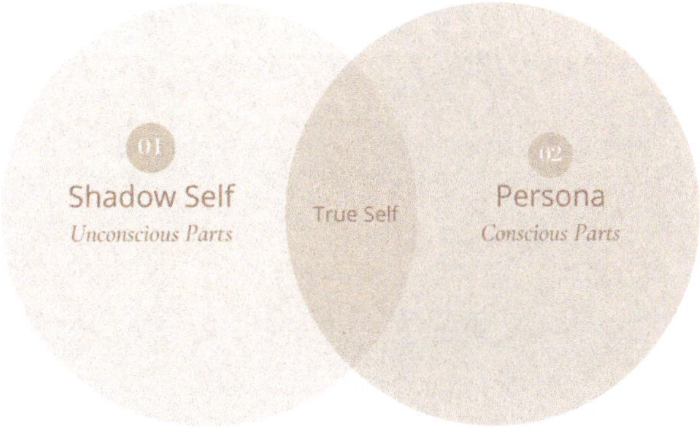

01

"Shadow Self" Identity

I have become aware of these blind spots:

02

"Persona" Identity

I want to be more authentic in these aspects:

PRACTICE

Inner VOICE

01 *My Inner Critic sounds like this:*

02 *It is this childhood caregiver's voice:*

03 *The cartoon character I chose:*

04 *What I change my Inner Voice to:*

INNER Child

01 *The parent's love I craved the most growing up is: (Mom or Dad?)*

02 *Who did I have to be to connect with this parent and receive love:*

03 *Who could I never be around this parent because this would have meant disconnection and loss of love or attunement:*

INNER Child

04 *This is how it ties into my dominant theme that's playing out:*

05 *This is how it ties into my unmet needs from childhood:*

06 *This is how it ties into my triggers:*

INNER Child

07 *This is how it ties into the voice of my Inner Critic:*

08 *This is how it ties into my lack of boundaries:*

09 *This is how it ties into my self-sabotage:*

INNER Child

10 *This is how it ties into aspects of my Shadow Self:*

11 *This is how it ties into the Persona I have created:*

12 *This is who my True Self is:*

PRACTICE

Boundaries

These are the new boundaries that I have committed to in order to reparent my Inner Child:

01

02

03

NOTES

01

02

03

EXAMPLE OVERVIEW

Shadow Work Process

This graphical way of filling in your awarenesses may help you create even more awareness of your patterns and how they play out in your daily life. On this page, you find an example to help you use this worksheet.

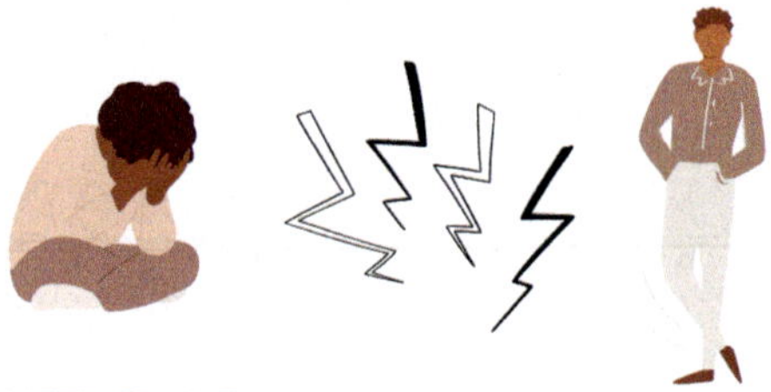

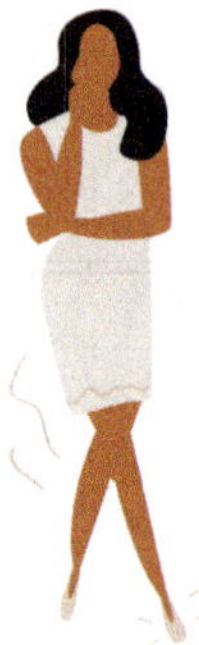

INNER CHILD
AGE: *3*

Dad
PERPETRATOR

ADULT YOU
AGE: *33*

01

Getting hit for disobedience

TRAUMA EXPERIENCE

INNER CHILD PROTECTING ITSELF

SHADOW WORK
= MEET NEEDS

05

When I feel helpless, defenseless, powerless I lash out at others in rage.

TRIGGER

02

THOUGHTS

I am helpless

I am defenseless

I need to protect myself

03

UNMET NEEDS

Feel loved and protected

Feel safe

04

COPING STRATEGIES

I need to control people so I can feel safe. I overpower others so I don't feel helpless.

07 MEET NEEDS

Choose safe people, remember I'm safe in trigger moments, do things my inner child enjoys

06 THEME(S)

Abandonment and Defectiveness

YOUR PERSONAL OVERVIEW

Shadow Work Process

This graphical way of filling in your awareness from your previous work may help you create even more awareness of your patterns, wounds, and coping strategies and how they play out in your daily life.

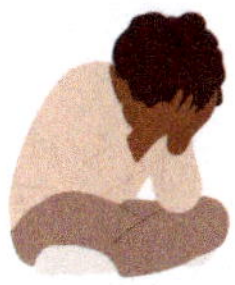

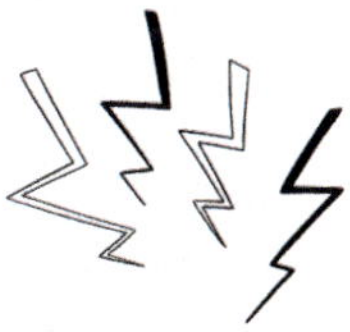

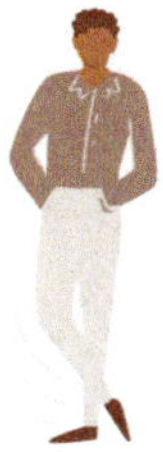

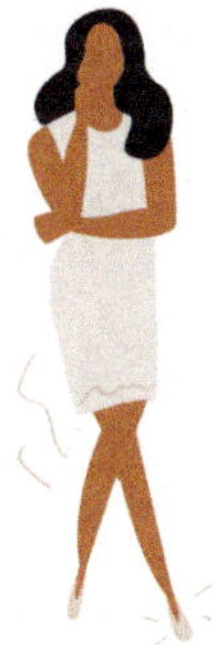

INNER CHILD
AGE: ______

______
PERPETRATOR

ADULT YOU
AGE: ______

01
______
TRAUMA EXPERIENCE

INNER CHILD PROTECTING ITSELF →

←→

SHADOW WORK
= MEET NEEDS

05
______
TRIGGER

02
THOUGHTS
______
______
______
______

→

03
UNMET NEEDS
______
______
______
______

→

04
COPING STRATEGIES
______
______
______
______

07 MEET NEEDS ______
______

06 THEME(S) ______
______

DAILY PRACTICE

Shadow Work Tracker

WHAT FELT CHALLENGING?

CONCLUSION:

TRIGGERS / THOUGHTS / THEMES

01

02

03

WHAT FELT LIBERATING?

CONCLUSION:

THOUGHTS / CHOICES / AWARENESS

01

02

03

EXERCISE

Challenging the Persona

We like to portray ourselves in a good light and showcase the praise-worthy parts of ourselves. We think of ourselves as a "good person," don't we? Maybe because we had to be the "good girl/boy" when we were young and it stuck as an identity. This amplified the split between our Persona and our Shadow Self. But as you now know these disowned parts will always be reflected to us and will usher themselves into our lives to be seen. Write down all your positive qualities and then try to identify the opposite within yourself. For instance, if you identify as a disciplined person, you're repressing your lazy part. The lazy part is disowned and hiding in the shadow. From there it is influencing your behavior and constantly challenges your disciplined part. It's okay to be lazy at times, then explore why you feel it's wrong.

YOUR POSITIVE QUALITIES	THE SHADOW SELF
✔	✖
✔	✖
✔	✖

WHY ARE YOUR SHADOWS NOT ACCEPTABLE?

What bad "thing" would happen if you expressed them?

PERSONA EXERCISE

Journaling

REALIZATIONS

TRIGGER EXERCISE

Active Shadow Work

01 Pick a person that triggers you

Choose someone you have a strong emotional charge around. It may be positive or negative charge, but usually, a negative charge will be easier to work with initially. This person may irritate, anger, upset, or annoy you. But they could also trigger feelings of infatuation or obsession. Do NOT choose someone who has harmed, abused or traumatized you.

---

02 Describe what triggers you

Write it out in 3rd person, "S/he triggers me because..." Write down all the qualities and behaviors that trigger you. Be completely blunt and uncensored. No one will ever read this. This is for you and your own growth only.

---

03 Dialogue with this person

Imagine this person here and speak directly to them. Tell them what triggers you. Ask questions such as, "Why are you acting like this? What do you want from me? What are you teaching me? What are you showing me?" Notice the answers you receive back intuitively as replies in your mind or heart.

---

04 Embody the triggers

Embody the person and the qualities that trigger you about them from step 2. Speak as that person, imagining you see yourself in front of you. Speak in "I am"-language. This might feel awkward and it should – these are traits you've been denying or suppressing within yourself. Write it down.

---

05 Contemplate your own expression

Take some time to contemplate this experience and what you have learned about yourself. If someone or something triggers us there is always a lesson to be learned. They are the mirror for us so that we can grow. They are an externalized part of ourselves, part of our Shadow Self. Write down what you've learned about yourself and what you are re-owning.

TRIGGER EXERCISE

Journaling

REALIZATIONS

EXERCISE

Light Shadow

WHO ARE YOUR ROLE MODELS?	WHAT DO YOU ADMIRE ABOUT THEM?
01	
02	
03	

Only read this AFTER you've completed your role models and the traits you admire about them! Stop reading now. Now strike out the names of the role models and write your own name instead. These are qualities you perceive in them because they are within you!

I AM:

EXERCISE

Light Shadow

Please complete the exercise on the last page first before you continue with this exercise.

I
List

What are my light shadows? List your traits here:

2
Feel

Knowing that these are traits within me right now makes me feel...

3
Express

How am I already expressing these traits?

4
Embody

In what areas can I embody them more? What would that look like?

5
Transcend

What do I need to overcome, heal, or acknowledge to embody them more?

SELF-PACED

Journaling

REALIZATIONS

EXERCISE

Belief SHIFTING

1 Identify

What belief have I recognized that I find limiting and want to shift?

2 Core

Get to the core of the belief. Keep asking "because" until you are at the core belief. "I am unlovable because [answer], I'm flawed because [answer], etc."

3 Admit

What is the thing I don't want to admit to myself? What's under the surface?

4 Truth

Ask yourself, is it true? Journal your first thoughts. Let it free flow.

5 Transcend

What do I need to overcome, heal, or acknowledge to embody them more?

EXERCISE

Belief SHIFTING

6

Release

Release statement: Now here in this moment the belief [name belief] is dissolved through all dimensions of time and space, past, present, and future, I am free x3.

7

New

Without this thought, what would you be thinking now? With it gone, what do you know now to be true about yourself, your life, and what you get to have?

8

List

What are your new beliefs? List them out.

9

Install

Belief Install Statement; I command and request from the highest realms of love and light to download the energy of knowing, understanding, and being of [new belief]. Visualize this new energy descending down into you. Expect to receive guidance and situations that help you heal.

10

Visualize

Visualize how you feel and act living this empowering belief. Step into being that person and this whole new vibe. Make it real. Connect to it.

SELF-PACED

Journaling

REALIZATIONS

10

FORGIVENESS

10

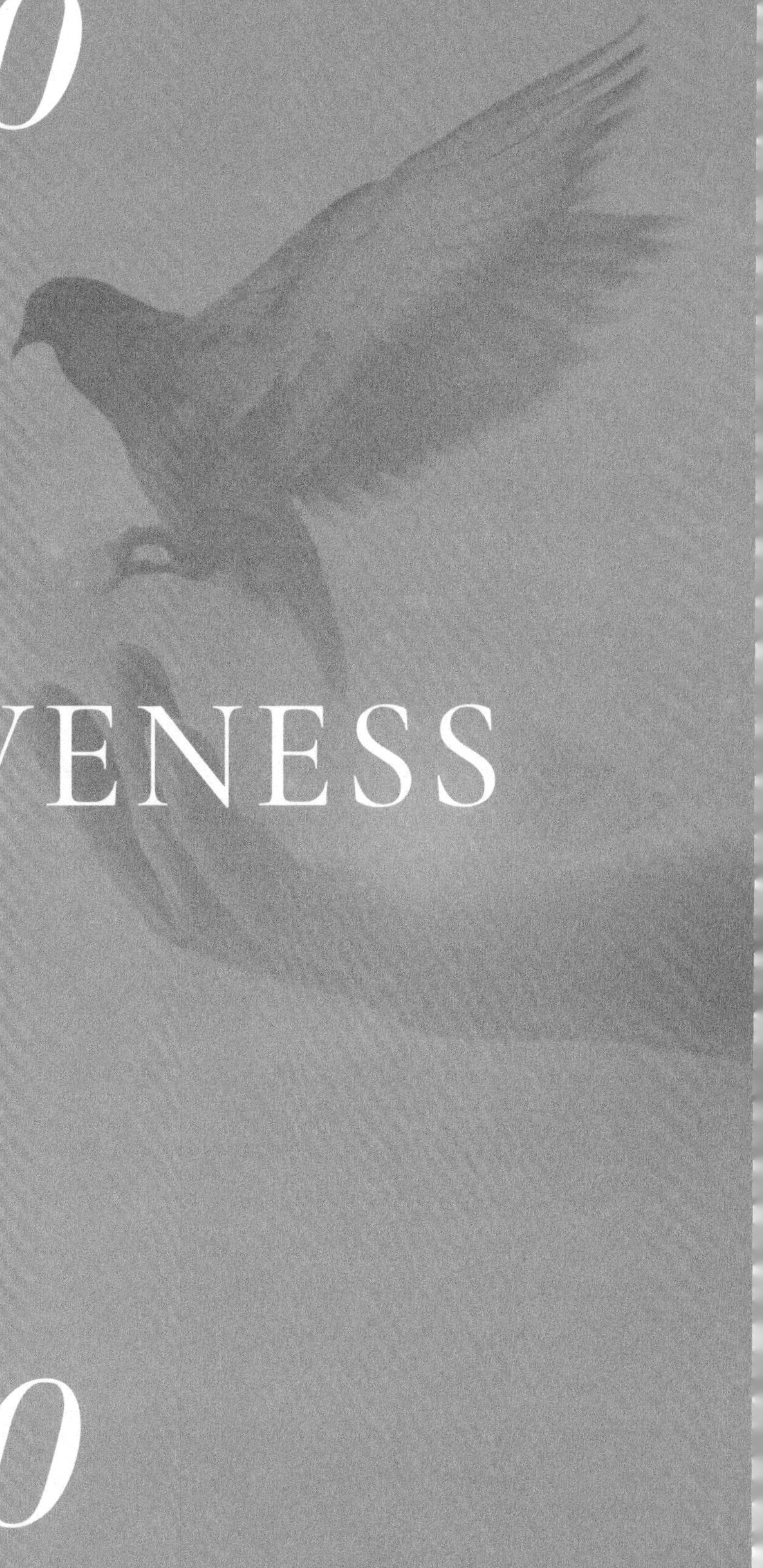

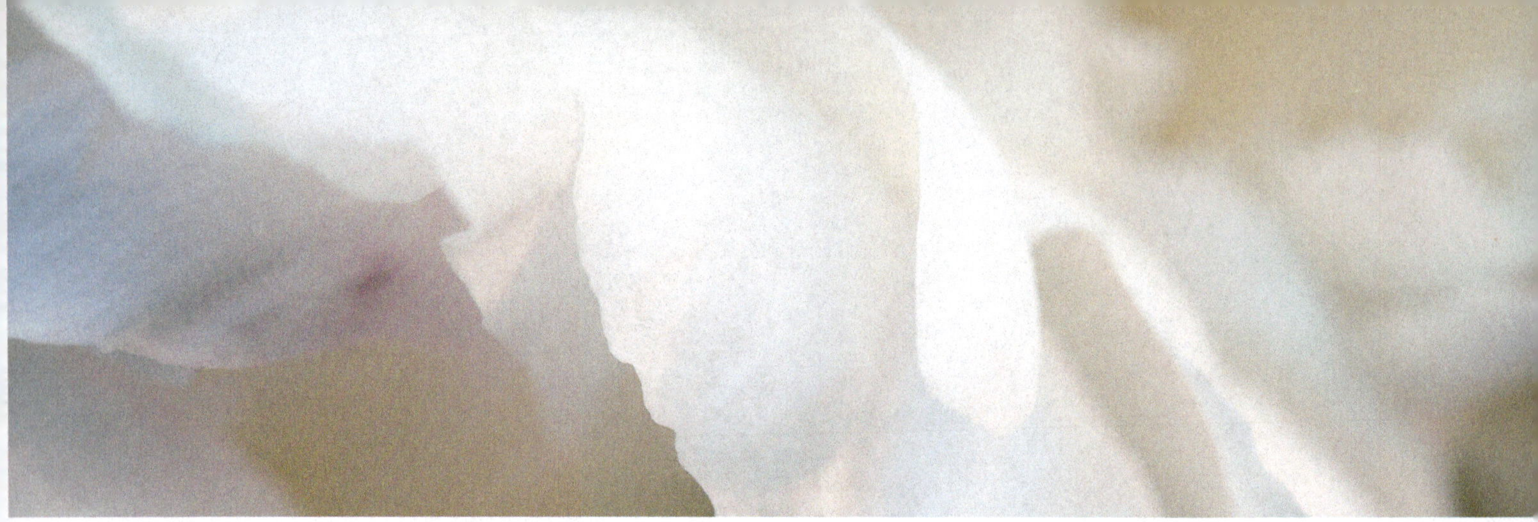

INTRODUCTION

10

Forgiveness

One of the most potent healing acts we can offer ourselves is forgiveness. When we forgive we release heavy energies that have weighed us down - whether we realize it or not. A lot of people carry guilt and shame around their shadow parts or past actions that were deemed "wrong."

We also hold on to resentments and grudges about people in our lives that we believe have wronged us. Resentment, guilt, and shame toward ourselves and others imprison us emotionally and energetically. They hold us captive in the past and keep us from liberating our energy and stepping into a more empowering future. We simply don't allow ourselves to be happy, thriving, and abundant.

Maybe you've heard the saying that holding on to resentment is like drinking poison and expecting the other person to die. Forgiveness is a process we do for ourselves and our personal growth. It is not about agreeing with what anyone else has done. They are responsible for their actions and the consequences of their actions. But we can free *ourselves* from these past experiences and choose to grow beyond them so they no longer impact our lives now.

On the next page, I offer you a Hawaiian forgiveness process that has worked well for me and my clients. You can use this process in two variants:

1. Visualize a person for forgiveness
2. Visualize yourself for self-forgiveness

One of the heaviest burdens is carrying the guilt for past actions. Often grief and loss can bring up a lot of guilt. Remember you did the best you could with what you knew and had available at the moment. You used your internal and external resources in the best way you could with your level of awareness and consciousness at the time. If you had known how the story continues you may have acted differently. It's okay. You deserve forgiveness too. Most likely this person would want you to heal and release yourself from your burdens.

Forgiving yourself as well as others doesn't mean forgetting what happened or allowing toxic people back into our lives. It means putting the burden of unforgiveness down and putting good boundaries into place so that we can move forward freely in our lives. We simply decide that the past, as well as that person, no longer has any power in our lives and we are free to be who we desire to be beyond any past trauma, pain, shame, or guilt.

Please do NOT use this process if you have experienced abuse and trauma with a person. It may bring up emotions that you can't process by yourself, choose professional help instead.

If you'd like to be guided through this process in meditation, you can use my free Ho'oponopono-inspired Forgiveness Meditation. Being held through this process can increase the potency of your transformation.

Guided Forgiveness Meditation

Use my guided Forgiveness Meditation feat. theta brainwaves for deep relaxation

LISTEN ON SPOTIFY

LISTEN ON YOUTUBE

Ho'oponopono

Forgiveness Process

Do NOT use for trauma or abuse!

01 *Opening*

Close your eyes and visualize the person sitting in front of you. Notice their face and notice who they are beyond the issue you have with them.

02 *"I'm sorry"*

Out loud or silently say to them, "I'm sorry." Take responsibility for the part you've played. This can be hard when we feel the other person has wronged us but no one exists in a vacuum and we have contributed to the situation most likely through our unconscious patterns. Notice what insights you receive.

03 *"Please forgive me"*

Out loud or silently say to them, "Please forgive me." Ask forgiveness for whatever feels right – wrong expectations, projections, emotional outbursts. Let your inner knowing guide you.

04 *"Thank you"*

Silently or out loud tell them, "Thank you." Thank you for the lesson, thank you for showing me my own shadows, thank you for holding space for this energy. Allow your truth to surface.

05 *"I love you"*

Say silently or out loud, "I love you." There is an idea that says the people we have the most issues with love us the most because they offer themselves for this difficult polarity. Whether this is true or not, we all come from one source energy and are walking each other home. Maybe you can see universal love or personal love beyond the conflict.

06 *Closing*

Visualize or imagine any energy you have activated in this process to drop out of your energy field and into the core of the earth for transmutation.

Journaling

REALIZATIONS

Journal PROMPTS

01 *Who do I feel has wronged me and what did they do? Describe it below.*

02 *How do I feel about it all? Describe your emotions in detail and don't be superficial here. Use the "Wheel of Feelings" to help you articulate what is alive for you emotionally.*

03 *Why do I feel this way about it? Explain in more detail.*

Journal PROMPTS

04 *How should this situation or experience have gone in my mind if it was "right"? Explore your expectations below.*

05 *Why haven't I let this go yet? What am I getting from holding on to this resentment? Is there some benefit (venting, being a victim, validation, etc.) I'm getting from holding on to this?*

06 *In what situations may I have treated others in a similar way? And how has this situation played out before for me? Write down why you think that could be happening.*

Journal PROMPTS

07 *Who would I be without this resentment? What do I need to realize to let this go now and be free from it forever?*

08 *What boundaries do I need to implement in similar situations in the future to make sure I am taken care of and feel safe?*

09 *What have I learned about my own shadow parts in this exercise? Remember we can only see an external reflection of what is within us. A part of us was available for this dynamic in order to heal. Journal below.*

Journaling

REALIZATIONS

SELF-FORGIVENESS

Journal PROMPTS

01 *What am I still beating myself up about? What do I feel guilty about? Where do I feel shame for my past actions? Describe the situation.*

02 *How do I feel about it all? Describe your emotions in detail and don't be superficial here. Use the "Wheel of Feelings" to help you articulate what is alive for you emotionally.*

03 *Why do I feel this way about it? Explain in more detail.*

Journal PROMPTS

04 *How should this situation or experience have gone in my mind if it was "right"? Explore your expectations below.*

05 *Why haven't I let this go yet? What am I getting from holding on to this resentment?*

06 *Is there a benefit I'm getting from holding on to this? Think along the lines of self-punishment, honoring a connection, not forgetting someone/keeping them alive, etc.*

Journal PROMPTS

07 *Who would I be without this guilt and shame? How would I act differently in my life? What new experiences could I attract?*

08 *What do I need to realize to let this go now and be free from it forever?*

09 *What have I learned about my own shadow parts in this exercise? What disowned parts need to be seen? What child-part needed healing?*

SELF-FORGIVENESS

Journaling

REALIZATIONS

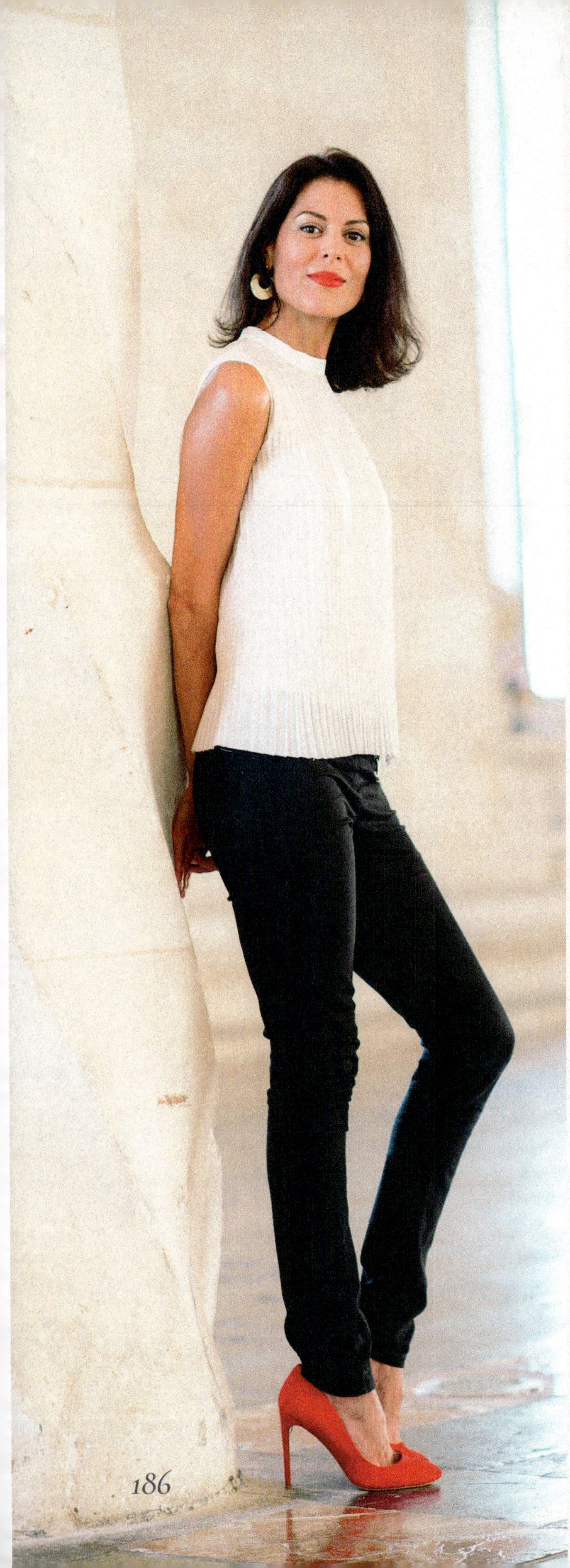

GOODBYE

Final Words

If you are reading this, you made it through the whole Shadow Work book. You are deeply committed to your personal growth and your ascension of consciousness. I just want to say, I honor you for that. It is rare for people to be so bold as to face their ugly parts and their deep wounding. You are doing well and I know you will keep healing and growing.

Do the best you can with your continued Shadow Work as it will be an ongoing process through life. You are well ahead of many others and give yourself credit for the hard work you are doing to end generational trauma. This is not easy but it will be worth it to find inner peace and acceptance. You are guided and you are loved beyond measure by the infinite intelligence and power that lives in all of us.

Sharon Kirstin

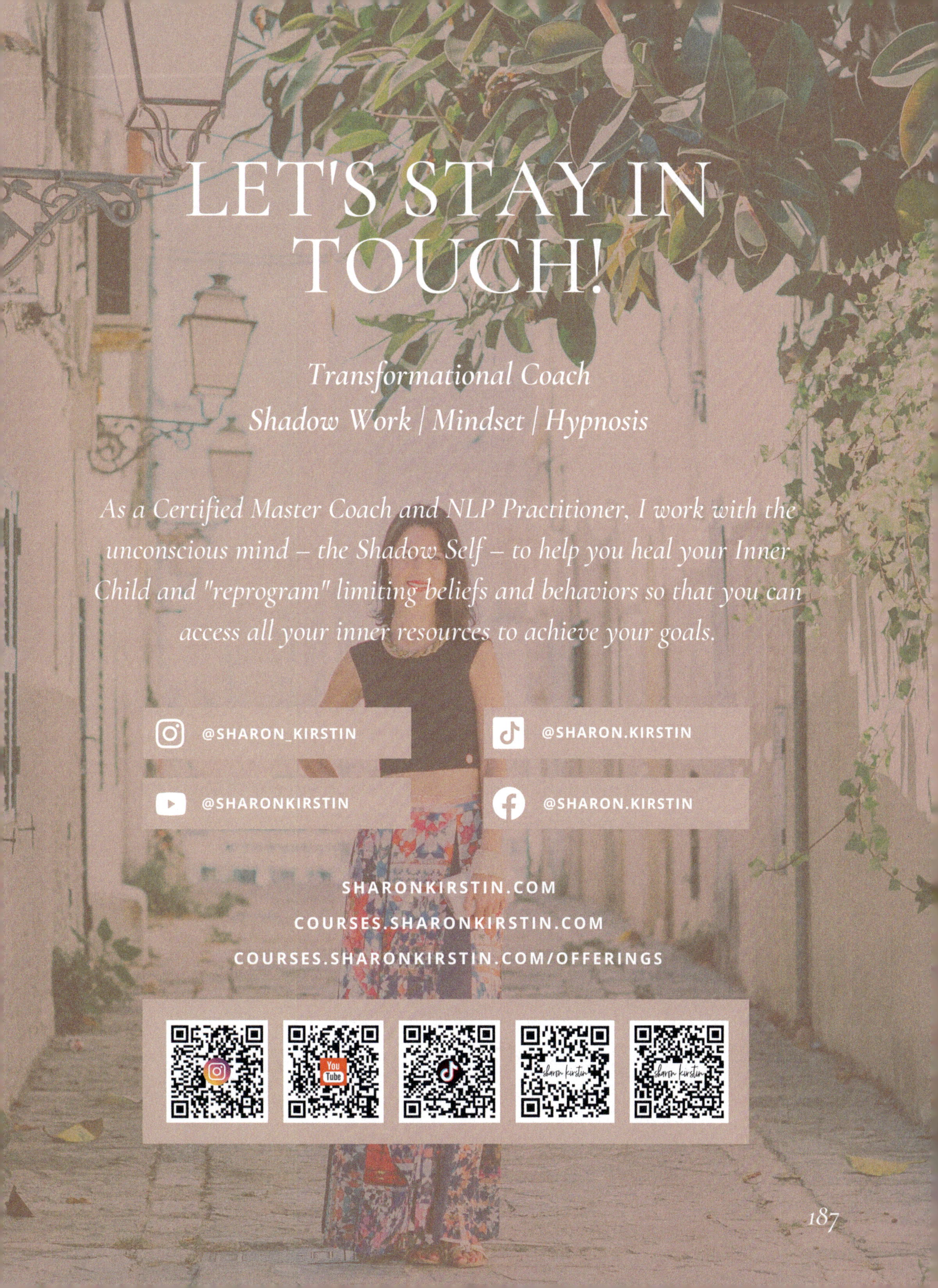

LET'S STAY IN TOUCH!

Transformational Coach
Shadow Work | Mindset | Hypnosis

As a Certified Master Coach and NLP Practitioner, I work with the unconscious mind – the Shadow Self – to help you heal your Inner Child and "reprogram" limiting beliefs and behaviors so that you can access all your inner resources to achieve your goals.

@SHARON_KIRSTIN

@SHARON.KIRSTIN

@SHARONKIRSTIN

@SHARON.KIRSTIN

SHARONKIRSTIN.COM
COURSES.SHARONKIRSTIN.COM
COURSES.SHARONKIRSTIN.COM/OFFERINGS

REVIEW & SHARE

Thank You For Being Here!

I really appreciate all of your feedback and
I love hearing what you have to say.

Would you please take two minutes now to **leave a helpful review on Amazon** and support others with their purchase decision?

Share a picture or video of the book on Instagram or TikTok
and get **20% off any course**.

DM @sharon_kirstin or care@sharonkirstin.com with your
video/photo link to receive your special discount.

Thanks so much!

Sharon Kirstin

12

RESOURCES

12

Free Download

3 MANIFESTING MEDITATIONS

WEALTH – HEALTH – LOVE

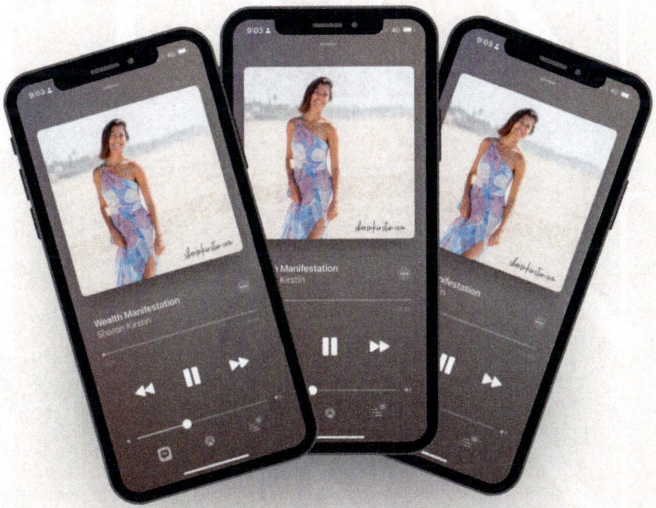

OWNLOAD FREE DOWNLOAD FREE DOWNLOAD FREE DOWNLOAD FREE DOWNLOAD FREE DOWNLOA

sharonkirstin.com/manifest

ladukie22 Your love meditation brought me my fiancé ❤️❤️
23m 1 like Reply

Sarah Rose ★★★★★
4 days ago in Westmount, QC, Canada
This meditation offers beautiful guidance and invites in empowering feelings that cascade through the body. I'm left with a feeling of gratitude for what I believe I will have ahead of time 💫

Ron gerber ★★★★★
3 months ago in Florida, USA
Never felt such an intensity and security with love until this. Thank you

Sara ★★★★★
2 months ago in Antibes, France
Very mighty! That's how I'm feeling now and that's how this meditation is. Thank you, thank you, thank you

Arkadiusz Ptaśnik ★★★★★
2 months ago in Birmingham, United Kingdom
That was powerful, thank you for a great meditation!

Cici Chapman ★★★★★
2 months ago
Truly, truly incredible and perfect for manifesting money and future goals!! 💖🙏✨

Monica Szymonik ★★★★★
2 months ago
I use this meditation each and every day. I've been meditating to this daily for 2 months. I love Sharon's style and pace. I love the application of the dimensions and archangel Ariel

Kristin Morin ★★★★★
last month in Millbury, MA, USA
Great manifesting meditation. I will definitely be listening again!

Grace Mueller ★★★★★
28 days ago in Blumenau, Brazil
One of the best in my opinion. Great guide. Great meditation

Liz DeLorme Garfield ★★★★★
last month
Supportive and relaxing

Erick Salgado ★★★★★
11 days ago in Franklin, TN, USA
Great visual guidance!

David Burk ★★★★★
10 days ago in Las Vegas, NV, USA
Excellent! Thank you

Charlotte ★★★★★
29 days ago
Love this meditation! Very easy to follow and listen to. This will be a part of our regular daily practise. Thank you!

Carol ★★★★★
18 days ago in New York, New York
Never realized how much negative self talk I practiced. Thank you for this meditation that left me happier and healthier mentally and physically 🙏😘

Alicia McDermott ★★★★★
2 months ago in Quito, Ecuador
Thank you! A very relaxing, heart-opening meditation.

Søny ★★★★★
2 days ago in Georgetown, Guyana
Very enlightening!
Gratitude 🙏

Candice Connor ★★★★★
29 days ago
I really enjoyed this meditation. The visualization techniques are really wonderful and I could see my dreams & desires that will manifest in the future so clearly.

Jacqueline symons ★★★★★
3 months ago in Vancouver, Canada
Beautiful, soothing and heart-expanding. Will be repeating often. Thank you 🙏✨💖

COURSES.SHARONKIRSTIN.COM

SELF-PACED COURSES

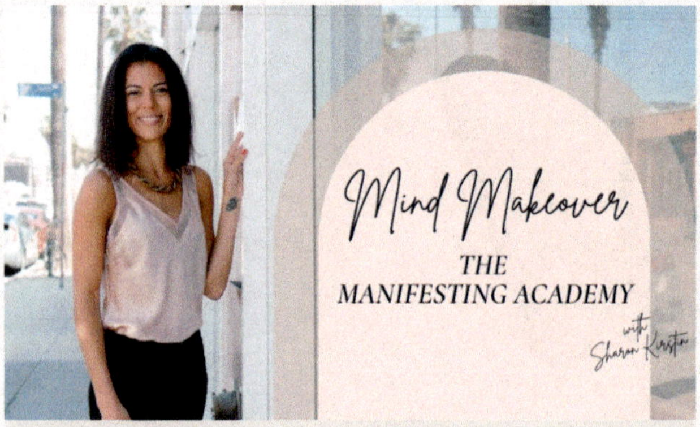

Mind Makeover

Deep dive into deconditioning your mind from limiting beliefs and unlock your next level of manifestation power.

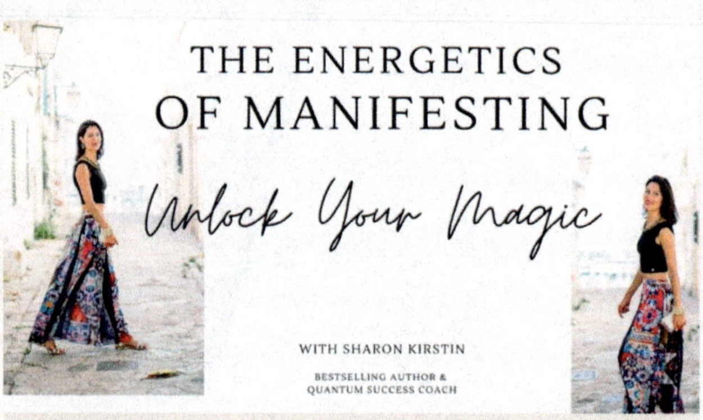

Energetics of Manifesting

Your Chakras, the Hermetic Principles (Universal Law) and the Manifesting Process play together, learn how in this course.

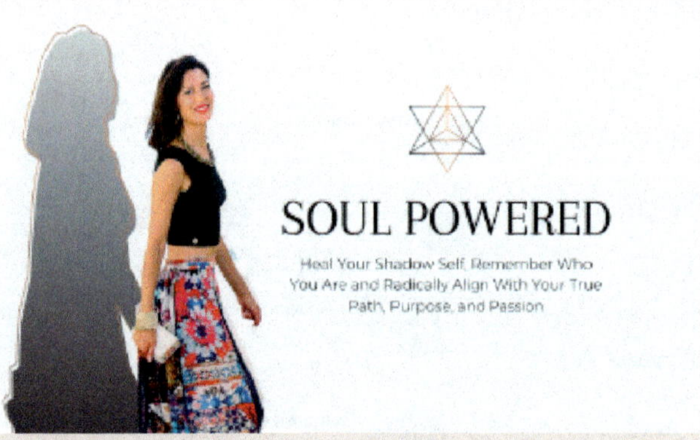

Soul Powered

14 daily inner work prompts for gentle Shadow Work to help you remember who you are and align with your authentic path.

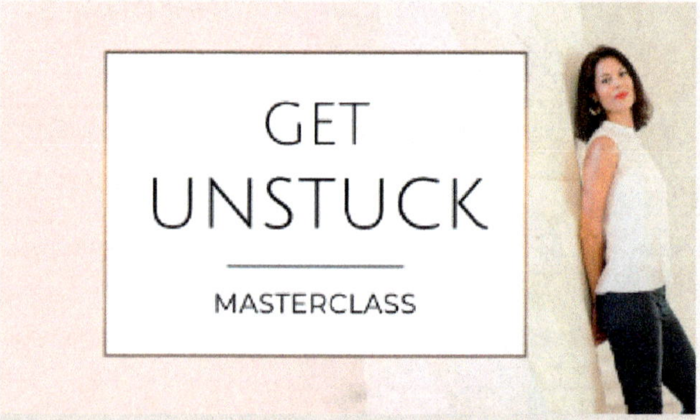

Get Unstuck

Ever put too much pressure on yourself, felt behind, compared yourself to others, or were afraid to be seen? This one is for you.

COURSES.SHARONKIRSTIN.COM

SELF-PACED COURSES

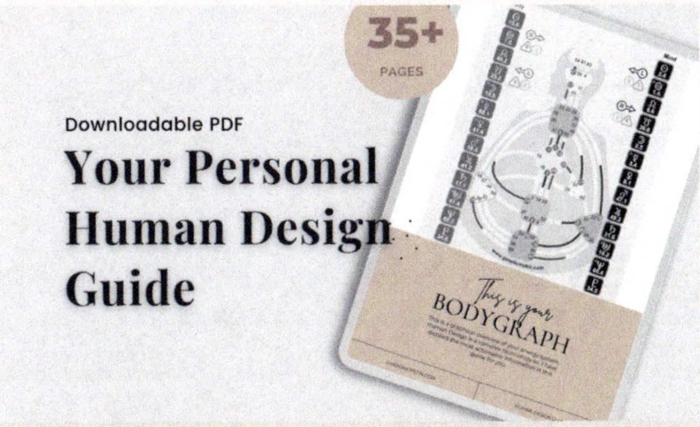

Human Design Guide

Your 40+ page Human Design chart analysis in a stylish eBook format reveals who you are designed to be in this life so you can manifest your full potential.

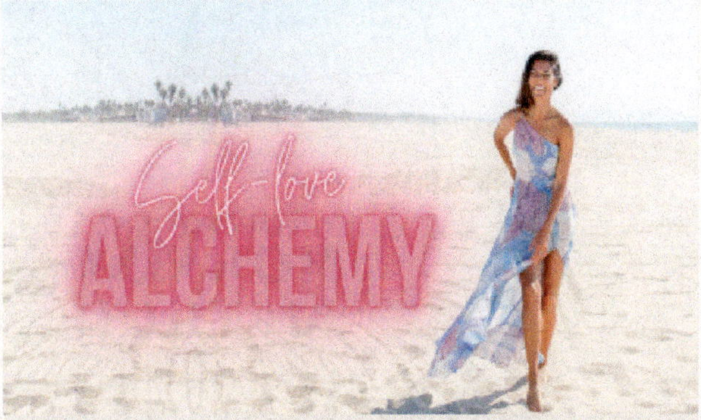

Self-Love Alchemy

21 Days To Love Yourself To Success: Quit The Hustle. Charge Your Worth. You deserve success, love, and happiness.

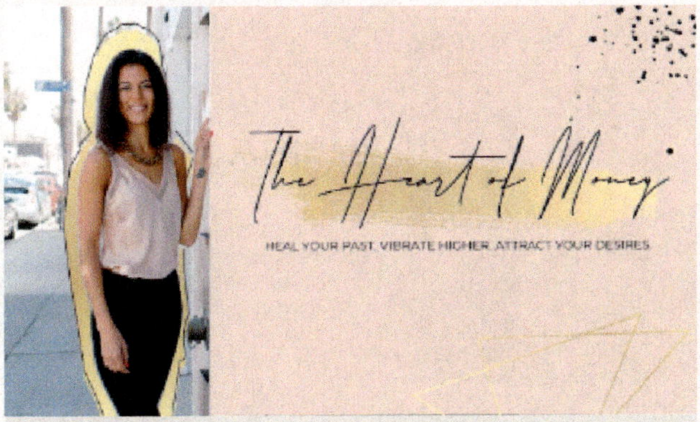

The Heart of Money

If you've ever struggled to ask for money for your gifts or you've doubted how much your gifts are worth, then this one is for you...

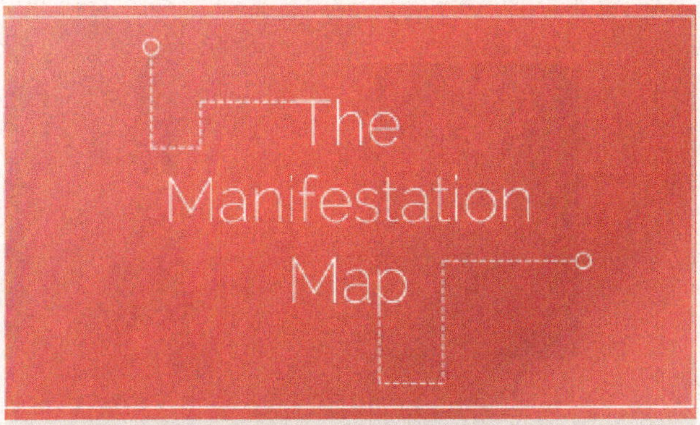

The Manifestation Map

4-Week practical course in energy mastery to become a vibrational match for your dream life.

COURSES.SHARONKIRSTIN.COM

SELF-PACED COURSES

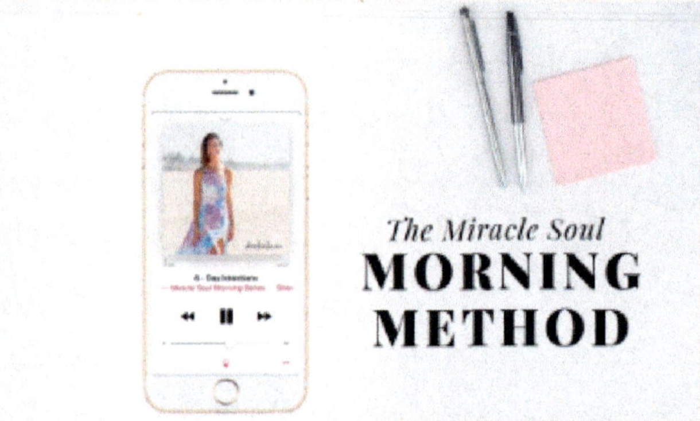

Morning Routine

Prime yourself each day to manifest your dreams and know your aligned action to take. Tried and tested – simply press play.

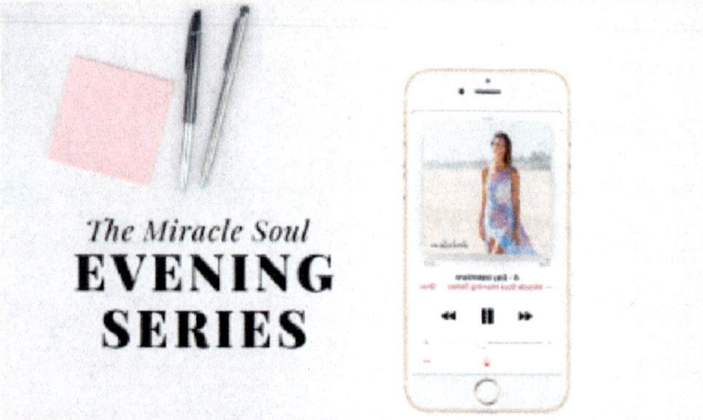

Evening Routine

3 essential elements in a strategically sequenced structure to release "icky" energies from the day so you can realign.

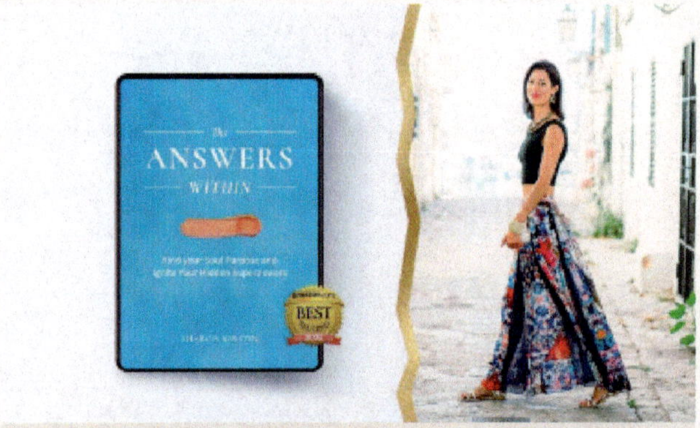

Best Selling Book Bundle

My book "The Answers Within", its exclusive companion workbook, spiritual practice planner, and Intuition Sleep Hypnosis.

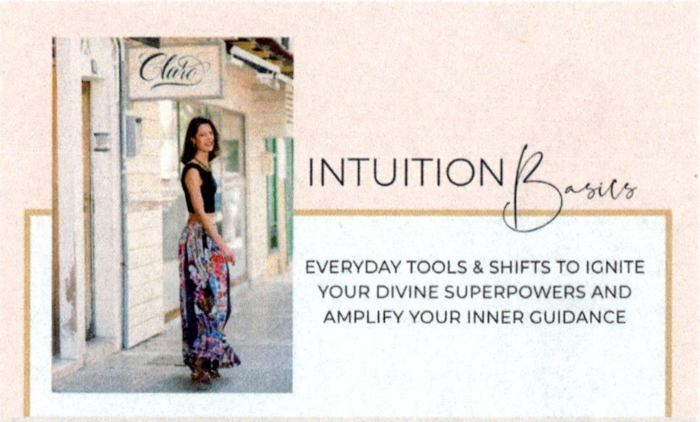

Intuition Basics

If you've ever wondered if you have special "spidey-senses" and how you can "turn them on", this is for you...

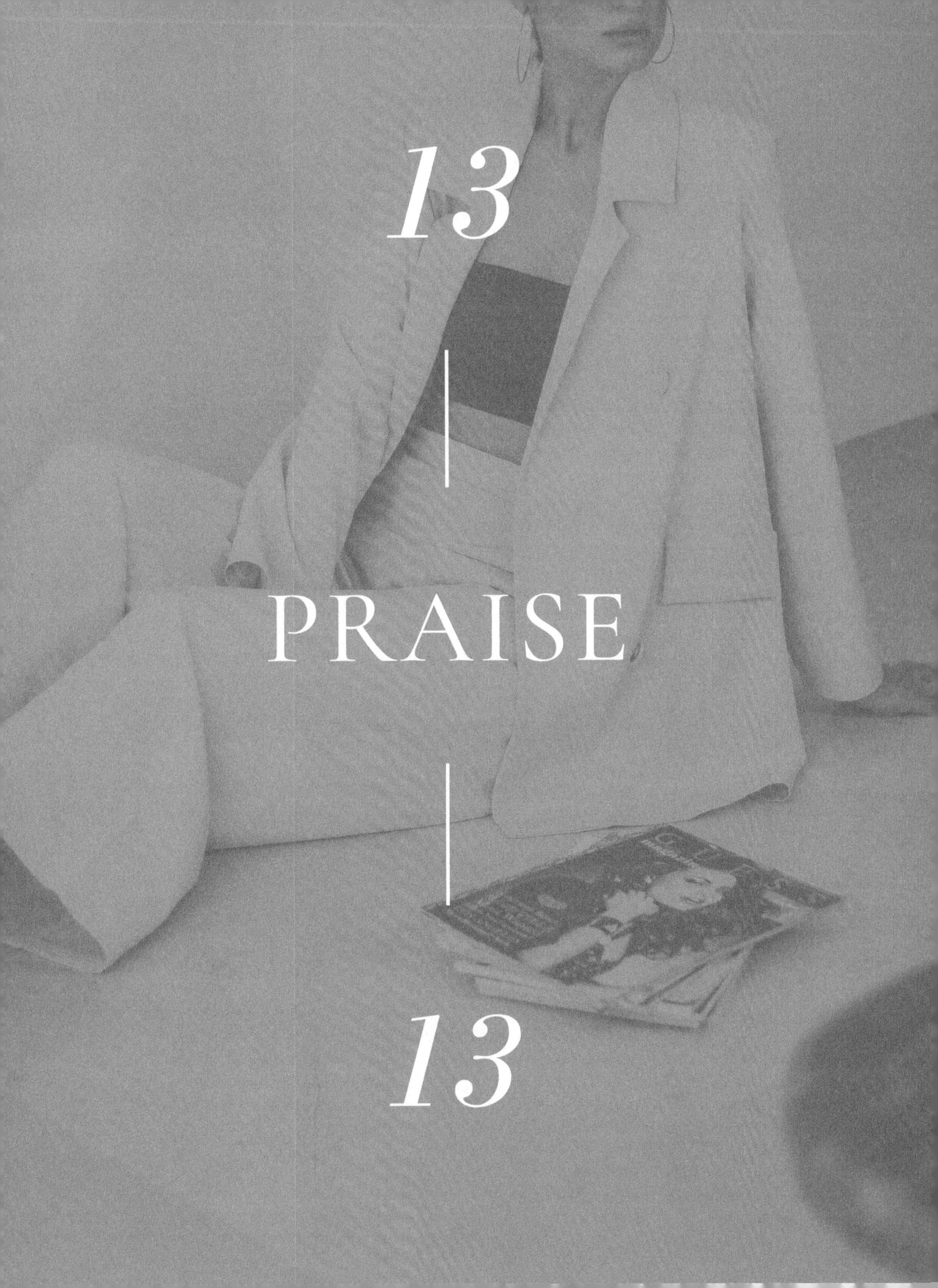

13

PRAISE

13

Testimonials

PRIVATE COACHING

★★★★★

"Sharon not only helped me transform in such a short period of time but empowered me to be able to continue the work on my own. I live every day fearlessly and unapologetic. I make my own decisions and not from my own mind's chatter or from fear and conditioning but from my truest self." –EMANUELA ELIAS

★★★★★

"Working with Sharon pushed me to do, feel, and think about things in ways I never had before, which has literally changed my life. Sharon, you helped me change my outlook from timid to confident, fearful to empowered, dark thoughts into light-filled life. I am forever grateful to you. You have no idea the impact you had on me." – LINDSAY LEE WILLIAMS

★★★★★

"I wish I knew how much magic I'd get after signing up. The decision alone caused a shift in perspective. I was so scared about the amount I'm spending on coaching with Sharon but it was unnecessary. I wish I had signed up sooner! If you feel the pull, then it means "Yes, go for it!" Trust that pull. Be prepared for the magic contained in working with Sharon. "Awakening" the knowing within and connecting to that inner higher self. There are inner shifts that cause ripple effects and long-term results.

★★★★★

"Sharon's coaching was life-changing, and critical to me feeling peaceful, powerful, and whole! Sharon's 1-1 NLP coaching, online courses, and meditations helped me amplify my true voice - the soft voice within. She helped me shed anxiety around self-worth, shift beliefs blocking me from financial abundance, and let go of fear about stepping into my power. I no longer feel alone, and I have given myself permission to receive all the abundance that is flowing toward me!" – CANDACE SUAVE

Testimonials

PRIVATE COACHING

★★★★★

"Wow! I can't say enough...a one-hour Discovery Call turned out to be one of the best therapy sessions I ever had (I mean better than any psychotherapist). Sharon's sweet yet confident energy truly resonated with me and she got to the core of what has been a lifelong mindset roadblock." – MARIELA ALARIE

★★★★★

"Sharon takes you from where you are stuck - and gently helps you oil the wheels of creativity and perspective, using advanced healing methods to help release resistance and promote a knowing of ease. If you want to create flow and manifest outcomes that are currently out of your reach, Sharon is the right fit for you. Best investment I made for my business and life." – SHEELAGH MARIA

★★★★★

"Sharon has a gift. She's one of the most connected and intuitive humans I've ever had the pleasure of working with. She has a fine balance with understanding the types of practical problems a tech CEO would face in the real world. This makes her a great teammate for any CEO, solving big problems in the world that is looking for more guidance, and wants to take their energy and overall game to the next level." – TOM LEV

★★★★★

"Sharon has a wonderful and warm way of being present for her clients, guiding them easily back to themselves and toward The Power Within. Sharon's ability to encourage, as well as shine a light forward is remarkable as you experience it in all its quiet and resolute power. I would recommend Sharon's coaching to anyone who seeks greater clarity and greater truth in understanding and working with the unseen energy we possess and how to harness and direct that energy for our own and others' greatest good." – RALPH ADAMO

Testimonials

MONEY RELATIONSHIP RESET

★★★★★

"I have experienced incredible changes working with Sharon regularly. What I loved about this Money Relationship Reset was how *quickly* the shifts came. It's been truly unbelievable. In a matter of four weeks, I went from a super anxious and unstable relationship with money to a calm and secure relationship with it. Fear around bigger money investments has dissipated. I have detached from fear, greed, and survival-based feelings around money. If you're on the fence about working on your money relationship with Sharon, please just allow the doubts, fears, or anxieties around investing in this course to just pass right on through. The peace I have in my relationship with money is invaluable and ANY time I've invested with Sharon it's returned 10-fold and this time was no different." – EMANUELA ELIAS

★★★★★

"Everything about how I view money has changed. I went from feeling that I am bad with money to trusting money to be there for me. From feeling like I need to lower my desires and ambitions to now feeling worthy of absolutely everything I desire. I have secured a 5 figure contract and now see those pieces of work as 'easy'. The best bit of working with Sharon was shifting the deep patterning which had affected me. I realized a lot of work around my money mindset had been too surface level before. She was able to deliver very powerful visualisations for me and guided me through blocks to see things differently. I now trust that money will be there for me, it's so empowering!" – JANE

Testimonials

MONEY RELATIONSHIP RESET

★★★★★

"If I had a message for others it would be this: Money is love. Feeling a deep love for money felt absolutely impossible only a few weeks ago before working with Sharon I was imbalanced, doubting my offers, in a low vibration, frustrated, stuck, and not believing in myself. Money didn't mean much to me, it felt wrong and bad, useless. I am especially grateful for the processes we went through to heal my money issues because they were truly transformational. As a result my money relationship changed drastically: I now have more self-love, I feel a deep love for money, I am more connected to everything, more compassionate, more effortless, more secure and I believe in myself. I feel mutual love and acceptance with money and worthy of having more than enough. I recommend you try her money relationship work!" – Isabelle Heymanns

★★★★★

"When I signed up for Money Relationship Reset, I was feeling directionless, wanting to do many things but not finishing things, which made things difficult to move forward. But now I have more job and business opportunities coming to me, as well as to my partner. Money is rubbing off in the relationship! I now believe that I am money, I vibrate money and I am provided for 24/7. Working with Sharon's program shed light on so many issues that I was unaware of. I thought I had done enough healing but working with Sharon opened another aspect o healing, especially inner child issues. I liked the methods she used to uncover, release, heal, and eventually integrate. Thank you so much, Sharon! I highly recommend this program. Very happy I took it, enjoy quantum leaping!"
– EDEN CARPEDIEM

Testimonials

MIND MAKEOVER

ONLINE COURSE

★★★★★

"The Mind Makeover was masterful at creating a roadmap that kept me accountable to my vibrational frequency and what I desire to attract. The guided inner work has helped me feel less triggered and reactive by my emotions. What a relief! Sharon's course shifted my resistance and reminded me to let my desires come to me. Once I surrendered the belief systems (BS) that were weighing me down, I manifested a substantial increase in my income and improved my family interactions. There were endless aha moments for me that lead to a deeper understanding of myself and for that I'm forever grateful! Sharon will make you laugh while guiding you to where you needed to go. How far is up to you." – ANGELA ORTIZ

★★★★★

"Sharon's weekly teachings in The Mastermind have blown my mind, the knowledge and insights she has on the Power of Attraction are incredible. I am absolutely loving the content! I look forward to receiving her weekly teachings and have often watched on repeat. I have learned so much about myself, how I have operated in my life thus far, and understand why I have manifested results that are not what I desire. Since joining it has really been an open-hearted and deeply connected space that has allowed me to openly share without prejudice. With Sharon's support, I am held to strongly believe that "I am not broken". I have increased my vibration by challenging old behaviors and patterns and am allowing my soul-led life more and more." – LYNSEY COWAN

Testimonials

MIND MAKEOVER

ONLINE COURSE

★★★★★

"I first heard of Sharon from reading her book "The Answers Within." That started me on a path of self-exploration, I just knew I had it within me to create and live my best life. After trying just about every book, video, and course I could find, something was still missing. I wanted to be able to tie it all together and manifest the things I desired. None of them shifted my life like the Mind Makeover - The Manifesting Mastermind. Sharon's no-nonsense approach and getting straight to the matter have transformed my inner guidance as nothing else has. This course and Sharon's tools, guidance, and meditations have helped create profound changes in my consciousness that have helped me identify and knock out the limiting beliefs that held me back for so long. The transformation taking place in my internal world has shown up in my external life as well! Even among the chaos of our world in 2020, I feel a strong sense of peace and understanding. Sharon is a talented master coach and the Mastermind Modules are the highlight of my week!" – MICHELLE BLAZER

★★★★★

"One of the biggest aha-moments for me happened straight in Module 1 of Mind Makeover. The shift was nearly immediate and quite liberating. I love the community as well. After some time, you feel like family, learning from and cheering for one another. Listening to Sharon help me and others shift mindsets and perceptions is like watching unstructured magic happen as the tricks present themselves. It's just amazing!" – CRISTIANO ALVES

Spiritual Awakening is not a one-time event. It's a continuous process of realizing higher levels of truth. Keep going!

xx Sharon

Printed in Great Britain
by Amazon

31070095R00123